Effective Counseling
in Stuttering Therapy

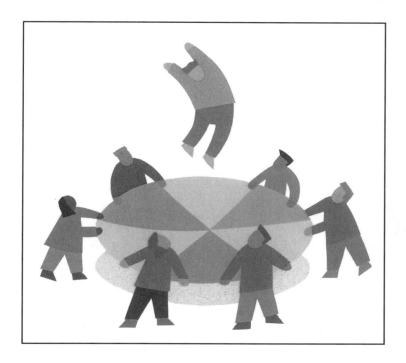

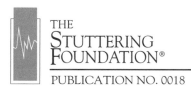
THE
STUTTERING
FOUNDATION®

PUBLICATION NO. 0018

effective counseling in stuttering therapy

Publication No. 0018

First Printing—2003
Second Printing—2006
Third Printing —2013

Published by

Stuttering Foundation of America
P. O. Box 11749
Memphis, Tennessee 38111-0749

ISBN 978-0-933388-52-9

Printed in the United States of America

To the Clinician

The original Stuttering Foundation book on counseling was written in 1981. The first edition took an innovative approach by including counseling as an integral part of stuttering therapy, and the authors hoped the book would help clinicians counsel their clients more effectively.

In the intervening years, the role of counseling in the therapy process has been more and more widely accepted as playing a crucial role in successful treatment.

In March 2003, a group of specialists in stuttering met for a week-long conference to discuss the current role of counseling in treatment of those who stutter: from parents of preschoolers to school-age children to adolescents to adults. Their chapters, as well as several from the original book, can be found on the following pages.

Your clinical effectiveness should be enhanced by careful consideration of the goals and processes described by these authors.

Jane Fraser
President

The Stuttering Foundation
May 2013

About the Authors

Eugene B. Cooper, Ed. D.
> Professor Emeritus, Communicative Disorders, University of Alabama. Editorial Consultant, *Journal of Fluency Disorders.* Author of *Personalized Fluency Control Therapy.*

Hugo G. Gregory, Ph.D. (1928–2004)
> Professor Emeritus, Speech and Language Pathology, Department of Communicative Disorders, Northwestern University. Editorial Consultant, *Journal of Fluency Disorders.* Author of *Stuttering Therapy, Rationale and Procedures.*

Barry Guitar, Ph.D., CCC-SLP
> Board Recognized Fluency Specialist and Professor of Communication Sciences at the University of Vermont. He is the author of *Stuttering: An integrated approach to its nature and treatment.* His clinical focus with preschool children who stutter is on parent-delivered treatment; his emphasis with school age children is on helping them stutter more easily and communicate more effectively.

Diane G. Hill, M.A., CCC-SLP
> Board Recognized Fluency Specialist. For 32 years, Ms. Hill was a Senior Lecturer and Clinic Supervisor in Speech-Language Pathology at Northwestern University. During her career, she developed and directed numerous preschool stuttering programs and contributed chapters on differential evaluation and treatment of young children who stutter.

Jane Fraser, Editor
> President, Stuttering Foundation of America. Co-author of *If Your Child Stutters: A Guide for Parents.*

Peter Ramig, Ph.D., CCC-SLP
> ASHA Fellow and Board Recognized Fluency Specialist, is Professor in the Department of Speech, Language and Hearing Sciences at the University of Colorado in Boulder. He writes and annually presents numerous practical application workshops and operates private practice clinics focusing on the evaluation and treatment of children and adults who stutter.

Julie Reville, M.S., CCC-SLP

Board Recognized Fluency Specialist and Clinical Instructor at the University of Vermont. She has worked with people who stutter in school, hospital and university clinic settings for 19 years. She is currently pursuing a master's degree in counseling. She is co-author of *Easy Talker.*

Joseph G. Sheehan, Ph.D. (1910–1983)

Formerly Professor of Psychology, Director, Psychology Speech Clinic, University of California, Los Angeles (UCLA). Former Editorial Consultant, Journal of Speech and Hearing Disorders, Journal of Communication Disorders.

Charles Van Riper, Ph.D. (1905–1994)

Formerly Distinguished Professor Emeritus and formerly Head, Department of Speech Pathology and Audiology, Western Michigan University. Honors of the American Speech-Language-Hearing Association. Author, *The Nature of Stuttering.*

Dean E. Williams, Ph.D. (1924–1994)

Formerly Professor, Speech Pathology and Audiology, University of Iowa. Fellow and formerly Councilor, American Speech-Language-Hearing Association. Editorial Board, Journal of Communication Disorders.

Patricia M. Zebrowski, Ph.D., CCC-SLP

ASHA Fellow and Board Recognized Fluency Specialist. Dr. Zebrowski is an Associate Professor in the Department of Speech Pathology and Audiology at the University of Iowa. Her teaching, research and clinical interests are in the area of stuttering, particularly as it occurs in young children.

Foreword

This book represents the culmination of a collaborative effort that started a little over two years ago. At that time, we (Fraser, Hill, Guitar, Ramig and Zebrowski) met to share our ideas for a videotape about counseling parents of young children who stutter. Over the next two years, we produced a videotape for speech-language pathologists (*Counseling: Listening To and Talking With Parents of Children Who Stutter,* 2002), and an accompanying User's Guide. Along the way, we decided to revisit *Counseling Those Who Stutter,* first published in 1981 and now in its seventh printing. The result is what you see before you; a compendium of approaches to counseling that includes classic pieces by undoubtedly the most influential writers in the field (e.g. Gregory, Sheehan, Van Riper, Williams), along with new chapters contributed by a more recent generation of clinicians, teachers and researchers.

Besides the obvious rewards we have gained by seeing our collective vision come to fruition, we have also developed an appreciation for the similarities and differences among us in the ways we incorporate counseling into our clinical work with those who stutter. As individualistic as we are in what we do, we nevertheless agree on this basic premise: That counseling is first and foremost about *listening to and talking with our clients,* and in doing so, helping them understand how their emotions affect their thoughts, and how their thoughts and beliefs motivate what they do. By recognizing this, our clients who stutter and their families can move ahead to problem-solve what *they* need to do to feel better.

In the following pages, you will read about various strategies for counseling people who stutter. Although we describe these strategies and how to use them — each of us in a different way— we all agree that counseling begins with listening to our clients and acknowledging their concerns and feelings. Throughout this process, we help our clients normalize these emotions. This allows the client or the client's family to formulate connections between their emotions and their actions; we can then guide them to discover alternative ways of behaving.

Although each of these chapters can stand alone as a resource for the specific population to which it refers, we encourage you to read the entire book in order to develop the most complete understanding of the process of counseling. For example, in Chapter 1, Gregory sets the stage by describing the importance of the clinician's thoughts and attitudes in the establishment of a strong client-clinician relationship. This discussion leads naturally into Chapter 2, in which Cooper presents the key features that clinicians should consider when planning a successful counseling experience for their clients and their families.

Sheehan's chapter (Chapter 3) is the companion piece to Cooper's, in that he discusses the feelings and attitudes that are common to those who stutter, along with specific principles of counseling that can defuse these emotions and help the person to re-evaluate attitudes about stuttering. The middle chapters of this book are devoted to counseling people who stutter and their families across the life-span, beginning with the parents of young preschool children (Hill; Chapter 4), school-aged children themselves (Williams, Chapter 5; Van Riper, Chapter 6; and Guitar and Reville, Chapter 7), teenagers (Zebrowski, Chapter 8), and finally, adults (Ramig, Chapter 9).

Effective counseling is an integral part of stuttering therapy, regardless of the age of the client or the severity of the problem. While the type and amount of counseling varies across individuals and families, the complex affective, behavioral and cognitive issues that make up stuttering demand that we provide no less.

Patricia M. Zebrowski

Table of Contents

chapter one
The Clinician's Attitudes 9
Hugo H. Gregory, Ph.D.

chapter two
Understanding the Process 19
Eugene B. Cooper, Ph.D.

chapter three
Principles of Counseling People Who Stutter 27
Joseph G. Sheehan, Ph.D.

chapter four
Counseling Parents of Children Who Stutter 37
Diane G. Hill, M.A.

chapter five
Talking with Children Who Stutter 53
Dean E. Williams, Ph.D.

chapter six
The Severe Young Stutterer 65
Charles Van Riper, Ph.D.

chapter seven
Counseling School-Age Children in Group Therapy . . . 71
Barry Guitar, Ph.D., and Julie Reville, M.S.

chapter eight
Understanding and Coping with Emotions:
Counseling Teenagers Who Stutter 85
Patricia M. Zebrowski, Ph.D.

chapter nine
Counseling Adults in Group Therapy 95
Peter R. Ramig, Ph.D.

Chapter **1**

the clinician's attitudes

Hugo H. Gregory, Ph.D.

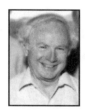 The relationship between the client's and clinician's attitude as interacting variables in therapy has received increased emphasis in recent years. Consequently, it appears important for clinicians working with those who stutter to have a greater awareness of the way in which their thoughts and feelings influence what they do in therapy.

The Clinician's Point of View

At any one time, we are the products of our training and professional experience. When we read a book on stuttering we digest and integrate new information. Every child and adult, including parents with whom we work, probably teaches us something new. Furthermore, when we discuss a client with another clinician, some aspect of the other clinician's perspective usually helps us in understanding our client better. In other words, we are clinicians in the process of change. A **cardinal attitude** we must have as clinicians is to modify our ideas as we give attention to new developments and new experiences. We should accept the professional challenge to learn new procedures and to evaluate the results we get when we modify therapy or parent counseling. Beyond this, we can generate new procedures for evaluation and treatment.

Clinician's Attitudes and the Client-Clinician Relationship

Clinicians' points of view about the nature of stuttering will influence their attitudes about the relationship between clinician and client. As we know, some writers are more specific than others about procedures for modifying the stutterer's attitudes and in discussing the dynamics of the client-clinician relationship. Thus, they also give more consideration to dimensions of the clinician's attitudes. What follows in this chapter is a discussion based on my experience as a clinician and a teacher.

Understanding the unique feelings and beliefs of the person who stutters or parent. One of the characteristics of a therapeutic relationship, often without parallel in a client's experience, is that the clinician enters the relationship with the attitude that each person with a stuttering problem has unique feelings and beliefs and that a situation should be established in which these attitudes are understood as well as possible. In creating an

...each person has unique feelings and beliefs

atmosphere that is conducive to understanding the client better, I suggest that clinicians ask themselves what kind of a person they prefer. Do they like a person who is genuinely interested in them, who takes time to listen, who seems to want to know them better or do they like a person who wants to impart information, to explain circumstances to them? We usually agree that we know more of the givers of information. It may be that giving information expresses dominance and giving direction is related to manipulation and control. Whereas we may view listening and attempting to understand as being indecisive and uncertain. For whatever reason, many speech-language pathologists seem to find it easier to be a provider of information and direction.

In my experience, there are three reasons why it is preferable to attempt to understand the client before we give information and make recommendations: (1) Most clients appreciate the interest we show and our efforts to understand their experiences and perceptions. It is important that we relate the information we give and therapy goals to that person's **unique experiences.** (2) What we do early in therapy establishes some of the basic conditions of therapy. If the clinician becomes too directive at the beginning of therapy, the client's main perception of the relationship may be one of student and teacher. In this case, we are less likely to get to know some important attitudes of the client. It is easier to move from being more permissive and understanding to more educational and directive as it is appropriate, than vice versa. (3) One additional reason the clinician needs to understand the client is that through talking, describing and explaining, the client will initiate a process of self-evaluation and reorganization of thinking. This process opens the way for the client to receive new information and direction. Thereafter, when the clinician counsels, suggestions can be related to ideas and experiences previously shared by the client. Furthermore, the clinician's accepting and understanding attitude serves as a model for client's self-acceptance of his present attitudes and concerns.

In counseling an adult, we try to understand how the person feels about his problem, what he thinks caused it, what he has done previously to help himself, and the like. In counseling with parents, we ask them to tell us how they came to be concerned about the child's speech, their observations, their reactions, etc. We listen and ask for clarification and further information. We reward them for sharing these perceptions and feelings with us. We are taking a client-centered approach and recognize the individuality of clients' present needs.

These statements about counseling in the early stages of therapy emphasize the importance of establishing from the beginning a certain kind of relationship between clinician and client. One of the most challenging aspects of being in a helping profession is the necessity to create a positive therapeutic environment for clients with differing cultural, educational, and personal backgrounds.

The most successful approach is to show clients that your attitude toward them is one of openness to their unique concerns and experience. Knowing this has always made me more comfortable in counseling because I have not felt that I had to immediately be "the big expert" about each client's problem, and more importantly, clients have told me they appreciated it.

Other attitudes of the clinician—be empathetic, supportive, and genuine. Time must be given to making a sincere effort to understand the clients' beliefs and feelings. The clinician expresses this understanding through verbal responses designated as warm, interested, accepting, etc. These verbal responses are expressions of affect. They communicate to clients in a specific way that you are sharing their feelings.

In responding empathetically, the clinician is identifying as best he can with the feelings or affective reactions the client is experiencing. He then communicates this understanding to the client. If clinicians have experienced sensitivity about some attribute of their own behavior, they can identify with the clients' sensitivity about speech fluency. If the clinician has experienced the feeling of seeing a child in his family seem frustrated when attempting to do a task, he can perhaps re-experience some of the feeling a mother has when she sees her child beginning to stutter. When the clinician expresses some degree of understanding to the mother, the clinician's empathy is reinforcing to her and should increase her willingness to explore her attitudes about her child. The clinician is saying, "I accept your emotional reactions and you can too! Don't be afraid of your feelings." At the same time, of course, the clinician is seeing that some of his own feelings can be expressed.

A clinician who does not reveal some honest feelings is probably not being genuine. On many occasions I have said to clients, "I have never experienced this particular situation before with other clients and I need to think about it." Even though I am a clinician who still stutters some, or perhaps because I am, I admit that listening to a moderately severe or severe stutterer makes me somewhat uncomfortable. Adults who stutter are especially sensitive to clinicians who appear to be wearing a false face. So, be yourself! Just as the client is an interesting individual to you, you can be an interesting person to the client. However, care should be exercised not to express feelings that could intrude on meeting your client's needs or be aimed more toward meeting a need you, the clinician, may have for counseling!

For example, as a parent experiencing frustrations with my own children, I have at times felt considerable need when counseling parents to talk about my family situation. While I have considered it appropriate to mention that my wife and I experience somewhat similar difficulties as those discussed with the parents of a stuttering child, I have never allowed the discussion to focus on the specific content of my problems.

You must see your clients' need for support when they come for help, begin to face their problem, explore their attitudes, and seek insight and direction. Recognize that this requires courage on their part and communicate this to them. If you think it desirable for them to analyze their stuttering pattern, in part by listening on a tape recorder, be aware that this is often difficult, and proceed at an appropriate pace. You may perhaps say: "It is hard to face up to behavior you want so much to avoid."

Providing information and giving directions. We recommend that giving information and direction be de-emphasized during the early stages of the therapy. However, from the beginning, every client expects some information, and it should be given in a way that will help them clarify their own beliefs and feelings. We have stressed that information and advice or direction will be accepted more readily if clients realize that we have demonstrated a clear interest in understanding their ideas and experiences.

In talking with parents, we may give some information about speech development from the babbling stage, to first words, to conversational speech, giving special attention to the concept of normal disfluency. We may talk about factors that precipitate increased disfluency and stuttering. We talk "with" and not "at" them. As information is given, the discussion approach encourages an easy exchange of ideas. I strongly recommend that all behavior change activity be related to knowledge we have of the client as a unique person, and in addition, that we continue to listen carefully to the client's expressions of feelings and change as therapy progresses. At first, the clinician may be more permissive and understanding, then more directive and supportive, then challenging with an element of confrontation, and finally encouraging of independence. These behaviors are timed appropriately depending on the clinician's evaluation of the client's behavior, feelings, and understanding. For example, when clients are experiencing new successes in speaking situations, the clinician can challenge them to do more.

Clinician's attitudes about themselves. If we wish our clients to have more realistic attitudes, we should be more realistic about ourselves and be understanding of clients as unique individuals. Likewise, we must attempt to increase our awareness of our uniqueness—our areas of self-confidence and our insecurity.

...understand clients as unique individuals.

If you are reading this book, you are interested in the problem of stuttering, but you could be a speech pathologist who does not wish to include those who stutter in your practice. Possibly, you would like to specialize with children and the prevention of stuttering. If you feel insecure at present about working with adults, then admit this, and, if motivated to do so, proceed to secure additional training. In any case, be honest about your present knowledge and experience or feelings about the problem of stuttering as compared to other communicative disorders.

Have you developed some self-confidence about your ability to use a problem solving approach to analyze and work with some of your own personal difficulties? For example, have you defined a problem, thought of several possible solutions, chosen one, carried it out, and then evaluated the results? Obviously, this is one of the procedures your client has to use in therapy, so you will be more effective if you have used this approach successfully in your own life.

Have you monitored your sensitivity to criticism, your need to rationalize about your behavior, or your tendency to project into others an attitude that in reality is an attitude you have toward yourself? Regarding criticism, parents and other clients will sometimes question what you say or recommend. Can you recognize that you may have some emotional response to the criticism or the person's manner of being critical; yet realize that you should attempt to understand and that whatever you accomplish constructively must take this criticism into account? Concerning rationalization, if you recognize and accept in yourself a certain degree of this, you can help your clients have a realistic appreciation of this self-attitude. Furthermore, you can evaluate with more insight and objectivity the way in which you may be justifying a response to a client, e.g., giving an interpretation in counseling.

Finally, an awareness of projection, the tendency to see ourselves in others, should help you to make decisions that are based more properly on the client's needs. To expand self-awareness, you should participate in self-study programs that help increase insight into your own attitudes and behavior. Being an effective counselor requires a lifetime of self-study.

Referral for psychotherapy. All clinicians working with those who stutter should be able to deal with the attitudinal and behavioral characteristics related to the frustrations of stuttering and the concerns of the parent of a child who stutters. However, some may need broader forms of personal guidance if their insecurity or inadequacy is more pervasive and interferes with their ability to profit from therapy. We should recognize that other specialists, such as psychologists and social workers, may contribute usefully to the understanding of a client's problem and appropriate therapy. In some clinics, this need is recognized by including a psychological consultation in the evaluation procedure. Other clinicians observe adjustment patterns during therapy and refer for consultation and psychotherapy as needed.

If we establish a situation in which clients are comfortable to communicate, we may become aware of needs that go beyond our competence. When psychological insecurities and conflicts not so directly related to the speech problem are expressed, we should be calm and understanding. However, we should immediately consider the possibility of a referral. Here are a few signs of the need for psychological referrals that I have experienced recently: an adult revealed that he was frightened by his feelings of hostility although most people viewed him as passive; another reported concern over persistent unhappiness for which there did not appear to be a reason; a parent expressed her bewilderment over the responsibility of caring for her children and use of appropriate discipline; finally, a mother revealed that her married life had been unsatisfactory for several years.

I then express confidence in the psychologist, social worker or marriage counselor, etc. to whom a referral is made and express the idea that we all deserve help from time to time in resolving questions we have about our lives.

The clients' success. Stuttering is cyclic in occurrence and severity and the clinician must plan to help clients understand that. In therapy and following formal therapy, provision should be made for coping with degrees of regression. This happens to some extent with other speech problems, but we should realize that transfer and maintenance require substantially more attention and time in stuttering therapy. The clinician who understands this can help the client have a realistic perspective.

If we are realistic about the time commitment involved, I believe the results of work with those who stutter can be quite rewarding when compared with that of other speech problems. Careful and frequent measures of speech in various situations and self-reports of progress help clients view the results of therapy more objectively. In this way, both clinician and client can be realistic about progress.

Sometimes in spite of our best effort to reinforce the client and maintain motivation, they will not continue their effort and results will suffer. But we will never find a profession in which we will not at times be uncomfortably anxious about our decisions and suffer some guilt feelings. We must continually ask ourselves whether we are giving sufficient thought to our clients and planning to meet their needs as best we can. Success is probably not as absolute and immediate as we and clients may wish— or that sensational news stories may imply.

Conclusion

Self-study is an active process in which we should be engaged throughout our professional careers. The resulting insight into our feelings, beliefs, and behavior and the way in which these three are related, increases our objectivity as we evaluate clients and make decisions about treatment. Our point of

...always remain open to new information and ideas.

view at any one time influences the way we perceive a client's problem. We should remain open to new information and ideas. Clients are viewed as unique individuals whom we wish to understand, with a need for empathy, support, direction and reinforcement, and finally, with differing needs as therapy progresses. The more realistic we are about ourselves, the more able we are to respond positively and constructively to our clients.

Chapter 2

understanding the process

Eugene B. Cooper, Ph.D.

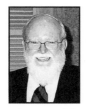 We know that people who stutter do not possess characteristic personality traits. As a group they are no different from groups of normally fluent speakers with respect to the presence or absence of psychopathology. We also know that chronic stutterers, like other groups of individuals with observable disabilities, may develop behaviors, feelings, and attitudes which impede therapy. Counseling is always part of stuttering therapy. For example, counseling is critical when therapy progress is impeded by 1) misperceptions, 2) emotional overlay, and 3) a disparity between the way the person who stutters thinks and feels about himself and his stuttering.

Misperceptions. Some people have very few misperceptions. They can accurately describe the way they stutter. They see the ramifications of their stuttering clearly and are able to accurately assess the reactions of others to their stuttering. Others are less fortunate. They may not be aware of what they do with their tongue, lips, and jaw during the moment of stuttering. They may think that their stuttering does not interfere with communication when in fact it does. They may think that their speech is so disfluent that every listener is pained by their speech when, in fact, most of their listeners are not even aware of their stuttering.

Emotional Overlay. Perceptions which directly affect our self-concept are more charged with emotion than those having little relevance to it. We feel strongly when someone challenges our feelings of self-worth but little or no emotional response when informed of an event with no relevance to our own lives or beliefs. It is difficult to get a child or an adult to work on his speech if he does not feel it is important. It is much easier to get a person to work on his speech if he feels his speech is important and his feelings of self-worth are threatened by his poor speech. In some instances, the stutterer's feelings of hopelessness and defeat based on misperceptions of the stuttering problem may be so strong that he may not even want to enter therapy. Misperceptions with little or no emotional significance can normally be altered through instruction, whereas misperceptions overlaid with feelings require a counseling relationship.

Disparity Between Thoughts and Feelings. The clinician should consider the lack of harmony between the way an individual thinks and feels about himself. A person who stutters may know he is bright but may not feel he is. He may be intellectually aware of the need to modify his speech but may not be emotionally committed to doing so.

Problems in the three areas noted above will gradually become evident to the clinician as the client's stuttering behavior and related attitudes are identified during the evaluation process prior to the initiation of therapy. Behavior and attitudinal patterns that may indicate the need for counseling will become even more evident as the client begins to make efforts to modify the stuttering behavior.

In a few instances, the client's problems in each of the three areas noted above will be of such a magnitude that the clinician will refer the client for a psychological evaluation to determine if psychotherapy is needed. In most instances, however, he will find that the chronic stutterer, although possessing therapy-impeding feelings, attitudes, and behaviors, will have sufficient intellectual and emotional integrity to benefit from the counseling process. Because the success of counseling is dependent primarily upon the client's ability to participate in the interchange of feelings and ideas with the clinician, counseling appears appropriate for those who are 1) in touch with reality, 2) capable of rational thought, and 3) have the potential for initiating and sustaining emotionally significant interpersonal relationships.

The Counseling Process

Counseling has been identified as the mutual exploration and exchange of ideas, attitudes, and feelings between a counselor and a client. In counseling, the clinician encourages clients to explore and to clarify, primarily by thinking out loud, their thoughts, feelings, and attitudes about their problems. Subsequently, based on the client's better self-understanding, the clinician assists the client in making his own decisions about what changes to make.

...counseling is a...mutual exploration and exchange of ideas, attitudes, and feelings...

Obviously, the relationship between client and clinician is a critical variable in successful counseling. Terms such as "warm," "personal," "supportive," "nurturing," and "friendly" have been used to describe this relationship. Such terms do not always describe the significant changes in client's feelings about the clinician, the client-clinician relationship, and the activities that typically occur during a successful therapy process.

The client may not **always** see the clinician as being "supportive" or "friendly." Many counselors go so far as to suggest that a counseling relationship in which the client always feels totally comfortable may even delay progress. They suggest that client self-evaluation activities (perhaps **the** critical activity in counseling) are stimulated most effectively when the client and clinician, through open and honest interchanges of feelings, attempt to resolve the uncomfortableness brought about by the client's negative feelings toward the clinician and the process. In fact, the counseling process may best be described on the basis of typical changes that occur in client's feelings as counseling proceeds.

1. Orientation. Counseling begins with the clinician giving the client an idea of the goals and a description of what to expect. The clinician notes how important the client-clinician relationship is and suggests that the relationship will undoubtedly be a topic of many discussions, particularly in the early stages. Also in the initial sessions, the clinician and the client begin the process of cataloguing and defining those behaviors, thoughts, feelings, and attitudes that constitute the stuttering problem.

Clients usually become more positive in their feelings toward the clinician and the process during their first session. This probably happens because the identification and cataloguing of stuttering behaviors and attitudes reduces anxiety. From a vague pervasive problem, stuttering has become more understandable, and the

...cataloguing behaviors and attitudes reduces anxiety.

stutterer is reassured. Now he can organize his thinking and focus on what to do. In addition, the clinician's description of the therapy process reassures the person who stutters that something can and will be done. These initial positive feelings become more important during the second stage of therapy when the relationship becomes more involved and more stressful, and the client becomes less positive.

2. Relationship. The second stage of counseling begins when the clinician and client focus on what to do. The specific aspects of the stuttering problem on which the clinician will focus will depend, of course, on his orientation to stuttering therapy. He may suggest modifying eye or hand movements during moments of disfluency or, if using a structured program, may begin teaching fluency initiating activities such as conversational rate control. Regardless of what specific adjustments are suggested, the client begins to feel pressure to make changes. These pressures naturally result in resistances that may occur even though the client appears to be making efforts to initiate change. For example, the client, finding that it is not so easy to modify the stuttering, may begin to deny the significance of the stuttering. In another instance, he may begin to intellectualize about the problem rather than to face the real feelings being generated by the pressures for change. In still another instance, he may simply give up, stating that he is incapable of doing the things being suggested by the clinician.

The nature and strength of the resistance that the client exhibits may give the clinician a clue about how therapy will progress and perhaps, about the client's prognosis. Of course, the clinician is interested not just in the client's resistances but also in the client's attitudinal and behavioral patterns that should facilitate change. Thus, the relationship stage of counseling begins with the person who stutters beginning to make changes and the clinician observing the client's reactions to his attempts. At this point in therapy, clients typically become less positive toward the clinical process and the clinician. Often, they are disappointed when they realize that the clinician can wave no magic wand to create fluency and that they must earn it through a long and arduous process of speech adjustments and self-monitoring.

The effective clinician is one who, understanding the inevitability of client resistances and disappointments at this stage of therapy, encourages the client to express these negative feelings. In fact, the skillful clinician uses these negative feelings to help the development

...use negative feelings to develop an open and honest relationship...

of an open and honest clinical relationship, necessary if counseling is to succeed. The manner in which a client's attention is drawn to his resistances and negative feelings is critical to the counseling process.

The clinician draws the client's attention to the resistances and feelings in such a manner that he sees the clinician as not being judgmental but as being open, honest, and above all, as having positive regard for him. To be successful in initiating an open and honest relationship, the clinician's comments must be based on accurate observations; they must be to the point; and they must carry with them the clinician's sense of respect and caring for the client as well as his belief that the client can make positive changes.

When clients understand that their expressions of negativism are accepted, they will express these feelings more openly and will begin to feel more comfortable in the relationship. In such an atmosphere, clients find that they can explore, examine, and discuss their feelings without the fear of being judged or misunderstood. The relationship stage of the counseling process is successfully completed when the client feels free to express both negative and positive feelings openly, to think aloud, to exchange ideas with the clinician, and to engage in self-evaluation without being judged by other people's standards. In such a relationship, the person who stutters will not only adopt the clinician's presumably more accurate perceptions of the stuttering problem, but also will begin to compare his own reactions to the problem with the clinician's. As the key factor in providing the client with better ways of viewing and valuing his stuttering, himself, and his fluency goals, the clinician may become a "reality check" for the client.

3. Adjustment and Planning. During the adjustment phase of the third stage of therapy, the client begins to correct misperceptions, to place his feelings in proper perspective, and to reduce the disparity between his thoughts and feelings. These changes will occur if the client has come to value the clinician's attitudes and feelings. It was noted that in the second stage of therapy, much of the time was spent discussing the client-clinician relationship, and there was an almost even interchange of verbalizations.

In the adjustment phase, however, the client does most of the talking and thinking aloud. The clinician simply reflects and clarifies what the client says. When the clinician feels that the client's perception of the problem and himself is relatively accurate, the clinician may begin the planning phase of the third stage of therapy.

In the planning phase, the client and the clinician establish mutually agreed upon goals. The degree to which the clinician takes the lead in identifying these goals will depend on the client's age, his abilities, the behaviors and attitudes to be modified, and the clinician's orientation to stuttering therapy. Obviously, young children will need the clinician's direction. The complexity and severity of the client's disfluencies and the extent to which his attitudes and feelings may hinder or help change, will also help determine how much responsibility the clinician assumes.

Clinicians favoring fluency shaping programs will suggest fluency goals already established within the therapy program being used. Other clinicians may help the client set his own goals after giving him a chance to explore various options for fluency control. Clinicians favoring a programmed therapy approach generally see the goal-setting phase as a discrete and brief phase of therapy. The clinician describes the program and, when the issues raised in the relationship stage of therapy are resolved, leads the client into the fourth and final stage of therapy. Clinicians who believe that therapy goals should be developed as therapy progresses continue the goal-setting activities initiated in this stage throughout the final stage of therapy. In the adjustment and planning stage of a successful therapy process, a key feature of the client-clinician relationship is the significant increase in the client's positive feelings toward the clinician and the therapy.

4. Application. The final stage of therapy might be described as being primarily instructional in nature. The assumption is made that the client, having progressed through the initial stages of therapy, sees himself and his problem accurately, has identified his goals and, to achieve those goals, needs only instruction in the application of specific techniques. The specific techniques used to elicit fluency in each client will, of course, vary according to the clinician's approach to stuttering therapy. Clinicians may approach fluency control by teaching the person who stutters to stutter more fluently by superimposing voluntary behaviors over the involuntary moments of stuttering. Others may focus on altering the stutterer's habitual speech patterns to maintain acceptable fluency in all situations. Many approaches have been found to be effective in eliciting increased fluency.

During the final stage of counseling, the interchange of feelings between the client and clinician stabilizes. Whereas a significant decrease in the stutterer's positive feelings toward the clinician and the therapy is characteristic of the second stage of therapy and a significant increase in positive feelings is characteristic of the third stage, the fourth stage is characterized by a leveling-off trend. In fact, in many instances, as the client prepares himself for the termination of therapy, a gradual decline in his positive feelings is observed. Such a decrease in positive feelings has been interpreted as an indication of his healthy withdrawal from dependency on the clinician.

A successful therapy process is concluded when the person who stutters has gained a better understanding of himself and his problems, has developed strategies for resolving the problem to the extent possible, and thinks and feels that he can maintain his gains without a formalized therapy relationship.

Chapter 3

principles of counseling people who stutter

Joseph G. Sheehan, Ph.D.

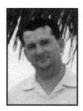 *Editor's Note: Joseph Sheehan, a pioneer in the field of stuttering and person who stuttered, understood the reality of the "giant in chains" complex and its disabling impact on those who stutter. This complex relates to an unrealistic belief that any accomplishment in life would be possible if only stuttering were not present. Dr. Sheehan was ahead of his time in using counseling principles as a major force in treatment. His understanding of fear, guilt, and shame and their relationship to stuttering was unparalleled. He was a highly successful clinician and researcher who devoted himself to the study of stuttering and its impact on life.*

All of us go through life meeting role expectations, or trying to meet them, sometimes succeeding, sometimes failing. When we fail publicly, we are shamed. When we fail privately in meeting our own self-expectations, we experience guilt.

Shame

Shame is an obvious occurrence in the disorder of stuttering, for the stutterer is expected to speak, and to speak fluently within normal limits, and fails to do so. In the process, he may exhibit behavior that listeners find mystifying and repellant, for talking

27

always seems simple to those who have forgotten how complex the skill was to acquire in the first place. To understand the disorder as clinicians, we need to experience these audience reactions, often by acquiring the role of the person with whom we are working so that we can know a part of what he experiences as he tries to speak but blocks instead. In the process, we may also experience a reaction of having done something wrong, of failing to do justice to ourselves and to our listeners. Like the stutterer, we can experience guilt, the private anguish that stems from the feeling that we haven't done right or haven't measured up.

Guilt

The part played by guilt in stuttering can hardly be over-estimated. It is likely that feelings of guilt lie heavily in the background of the onset of stuttering, help to maintain the behavior once started, and tremendously complicate the whole process of therapy and counseling those who stutter.

The impact of guilt on fluency may be observed even in normal speakers. When confessing something, or defending our own actions, or offering explanation under threat, none of us is likely to remain smoothly fluent. In those who stutter, guilt heightens fear, or multiplies with fear to undermine fluent word production. We reduce fear for the stutterer by decreasing his feelings that he is doing something wrong every time he stutters. This is what we mean by acceptance of the problem, of the "stutterer role," to a sufficient degree that the problem may be discussed, analyzed, and worked on in a healthy and open atmosphere.

We may distinguish among several kinds and possible sources of guilt reactions in those who stutter. Some of these are relived each time the stutterer blocks on a word, and may contribute to the mixture of shame, relief, and guilt many experience upon release of the word.

Sources of Shame and Guilt

1. Primary guilt refers to the constellation of feelings that preceded and led to the appearance of blocking speech in the first instance. For example, a child of two may have been negated and shamed so often that he is profoundly uncertain about trying speech at all. Speech reflects attitude toward oneself, among other things. If a young child has been made to feel that he is often wrong in everything, he easily comes to feel that he is wrong in his fumbling efforts to acquire the speaker role.

2. Secondary guilt stems from not fulfilling expectations to speak, once the stuttering behavior has emerged. The constant suggestions of neighbors and strangers to the stutterer to take a deep breath, to think what he has to say, to slow down, to try some trick—all these imply that stuttering is a simple problem with an easy solution if the stutterer will just follow the proffered advice. But usually, the stutterer has tried them all, failed with them all, and each reiteration of the suggestions merely adds to his frustration and despair. Morever, there is a role expectation of immediate improvement tied to these bits of advice. When the stutterer has to reject them, he feels guilty. When he tries them and they fail, he feels guilty. "When I Say No, I Feel Guilty," is the title of a popular book on assertion training. One of the book's suggestions for overcoming feelings of guilt and inadequacy is the technique of "Broken Record," a courteous but firm and persistent statement of what you really want. It is far more therapeutic to fulfill your own aspirations and expectations rather than those of others.

3. Audience punishment guilt stems from the client's realization that his struggling and grimacing speech is distressing and punishing to his listeners—or to his projection that his stuttering behavior is punishing to others. This is qualitatively different from merely feeling that you didn't measure up to fluency demands. Although there seem to be a few people so neurotic as to derive sadistic satisfaction from punishing audiences, they are not typical. Moreover, even those individuals can feel guilt along with the dubious satisfaction of having punished their audience along with themselves.

...we stutter most where it hurts most...

Research has well established a positive relationship between threat or expectation of penalty, and frequency of stuttering. We tend to stutter most where it hurts most. Ironically, it is often the case that the audience isn't nearly as concerned or as punished as the stutterer assumes or projects. Discussion of the stuttering problem with the clinician and observational assignments may greatly reduce the stutterer's guilt and concern about punishing the audience. Most people in therapy come eventually to realize that the damage they imagine they have been doing to listeners is like the premature reports of Mark Twain's death—greatly exaggerated.

4. Therapy-induced guilt is the fourth discernible kind, and it has profound effects on the course of therapy and the counselor's relationship to the stutterer. The implied or explicit contract with the stutterer calls for greater fluency, at least eventually. Every clinician wants to help the stutterer speak better—that's the reason the client is there. But there is a great hazard in premature expectations. Many a promising client, in terms of response to therapy, has bogged down over the knowledge that he is expected to improve soon. Where the pressures for fluent performance are scheduled ahead of the time the stutterer can get ready to deliver clinical failure and consequent guilt may ensue.

Readiness for change is a central element in all therapies. But not every person who comes, is sent, or is brought into therapy has a readiness to change. For example, many stutterers have well-stabilized patterns of retreat and subterfuge and aren't about to give them up without hefty resistance. As clinicians or counselors, we need to sharpen our ability to estimate the factor of readiness, so that we don't push when the client is not ready to move. At least, we don't push beyond his limits and receptiveness, or he may become so frustrated and guilty that he drops out or regresses rather than progresses.

Some degree of therapy-induced guilt is built in to the whole venture of therapy. Nearly all therapies currently in use call for the person who stutters to be an active participant to some degree. He has to do something besides just talk. Under these conditions, it is easy for the stutterer to feel guilty over not **doing** enough. If the clinician has unwittingly encouraged the common belief on the part of the stutterer that perfect, stutter-free speech must be the goal, the burden of guilt can never go away. Speech need not be letter-perfect or fluency-perfect in order to be acceptable. Even accomplished actors will flub at times. In fluency as in many other things, perfectionism is a self-defeating goal. Any persisting feeling on the part of the stutterer that he has failed on any dimension of therapy will tend to undermine the

—————————————————————
...perfectionism is a self-defeating goal.
—————————————————————

self-worth upon which fluency must be based.

5. Clinician-induced guilt. We have been discussing therapy-induced guilt, that is, feelings in the stutterer that develop from his awareness that he has not done enough, that he did not meet role-expectations he had set up for himself. The client may have some underlying mistrust of the therapist and the procedure he offers—and the feeling is often mutual. In this atmosphere lurks ample opportunity for self-blame and for other-blame. We have called the self-blame kind, therapy-induced guilt; it develops naturally and inadvertently. But some clinicians, deliberately or otherwise, induce guilt and shame reactions more directly. As an excuse for a program or clinician failure, they choose to manipulate the client's already strong guilt and shame readiness. After weeks or months of therapy with repeated relapse, they put an ironic twist on the idea of acceptance. Finally they say or imply to the stutterer, "After all, remember that you're a stutterer, and you might as well accept that fact."

Acceptance of the problem belongs at the start of therapy, not at the finish. It is the role that the stutterer must accept, not the old stuttering pattern. That is what the stutterer entered therapy to eliminate! If he should be asked to accept the old pattern, then he should not have been asked to undertake therapy. To promote "acceptance" at the end of the venture to excuse clinician failure or method failure is an outrage. We need not accept what we can change—and the person who stutters can change. If he had wanted to "accept," not for the purpose of enabling change, but in order to remain as he was when he came in, then he would not have come. When a clinician heaps blame on the stutterer at the *end* of therapy, then the client's hopes have been abused.

6. Timing as a source of guilt. As in any counseling relationship, the mishandling of the factor of readiness for change can lead to guilt and a vague sense of failure. Timing is crucial, for it reflects the sensitivity and competence of the clinician. An expectation to perform at a certain level at one stage may be less appropriate at another. Perfectly good procedures may be inappropriate depending upon the readiness of the person. For example, some discussion of the problem is endemic to virtually all therapies, even if only to spell out the arrangements. Some clients are just not ready to tolerate even that much self-confrontation. Even the discussion of the problem with the counselor may be painful. Skill in counseling people who stutter requires an ability to recognize discomfort signs, and to make sure that therapy-induced guilt does not lead to discouragement, low morale and premature termination.

Stuttering Coexists with Other Problems

Many other problems may coexist with the problem of stuttering, and the clinician needs to be equipped to help the stutterer with these problems, within reasonable limits. Becoming a person who stutters does not exempt anyone from becoming a person with many other problems. It should not be assumed that the guilt and inadequacy feelings often shown by those who stutter are entirely the result of the stuttering. As one example, a stutterer may seem depressed, and it would be easy for him—and the clinician—to assume that he is depressed because he stutters, or that he stutters because he is depressed. But the relationship of these factors cannot be assumed—they may be connected or not, or they may be connected but only minimally.

As another example, a client may be either hostile or pervasively anxious; but might he not be either of those things whether he stuttered or not? Such feelings might easily not be associated with his stuttering. Because hostility might be evidently connected with stuttering does not mean that it must be psychodynamically related in each and every case. The relationship of stuttering to coexisting problems is largely unexplored territory, and this question is left unanswered by those studies merely comparing stutterers with control groups. In individual diagnosis, the relationship of other problems to the stuttering must often await their emergence during the course of therapy. Problems that will affect the later course of therapy often fail to surface during the initial interview.

As clinicians we sometimes need to remind ourselves that we are treating a person, not just a case of excess disfluency. In some clinics, the stuttering group is called the "fluency group," apparently on the premise that fluency is the sole problem and the only goal worth mentioning. Many clinicians could facilitate the path toward fluent utterance more effectively by helping the person feel better about himself in all roles in his life, not just his speaking role.

A stutterer may feel ugly or lonely or unwanted or excluded from the mainstream of meaningful interactions with other human beings, and these feelings would all tend to contribute to the haltingness of his speech. But we cannot assume that he has these feelings only because he stutters. He might have them anyway. Nor can we assume that even a successful behavioral treatment of the stuttering would automatically remove all these feelings of self-doubt and inadequacy. By thinking only in terms of stuttering behavior, the clinician may overlook an opportunity to help those who stutter with other significant problems.

The "Giant in Chains" Complex

The client himself often thinks that if only he did not stutter, he would have no other problems, and there would be no end to his accomplishments. We have called this the "giant in chains" complex—the feelings that if only we did not have that problem, nothing else would be wrong. Awareness as clinicians of the overattribution of all problems to the stuttering may help us avoid the same illusion so frequently held by those who stutter, or by persons with any kind of handicap.

Nearly every stutterer has heard of the legend of Demosthenes, the Greek who overcame a speech impediment and became a great orator. It becomes almost a role-expectation. Yet we know that stutterers typically do not become great orators, even when they recover, with or without therapy. This is the "Demosthenes Complex."

The "giant in chains" idea is much broader. It refers to the overattribution on the part of the stutterer of all significant problems to the stuttering, to the handicap. If only he did not stutter, then there could be no limit to his accomplishments. Here is a defense function that can cause reactions of disappointment to the stutterer as he begins to improve. Unless we are aware of it, we may not realize that improvement brings many problems with it, and that there is a process of adjustment to fluency.

...there is a process of adjustment to fluency.

Respecting Feelings

In stuttering we deal with both feelings and behavior, with both classically conditioned and instrumentally conditioned patterns of response. As clinicians we need to be aware of the distinction between these two classes of response, for they require some different handling in therapy. On the feeling level there must be no right or wrong. If a stutterer feels fear or shame or guilt, then help him to explore those feelings, for they may relate crucially to his stuttering and to his attitude toward himself and others, and toward speaking in the world. On the feeling level, the "shoulds" and "should nots" must not apply. Otherwise the person who stutters will tailor his disclosure of feelings and attitudes toward what he imagines the clinician wants to hear. Feelings have a validity of their own and should be respected.

Some Principles of Counseling Stutterers

Let us concentrate on the attitudinal or feeling level, for it is here that the role of counseling enters most prominently. We may profit from emerging trends in counseling and psychotherapy generally, for we share the same presenting problems and challenges as do counselors and psychotherapists working with other designated problems.

A few specific principles of counseling the client with emphasis on the feeling level, to relieve him of guilt associated with stuttering and other things, may be stated:

- Create a relationship and an atmosphere in which he is able to express whatever he feels, without prior censorship. Help him understand that he is never wrong on the feeling level. In contrast, on the doing level, he has responsibility and choice.

- Make the stutterer as a person the focus of therapy, not just the immediate suppression of stuttering frequency. Help her realize her potential for growth and development and self-realization.

- Begin where the stutterer is, not where the clinician is. If he is fearful or overwhelmingly afraid to admit his fears, or feels guilty about them, give him running room enough to feel comfortable about what he feels.

- Respect her feelings—guilt, shame, fear, or anger—as having an intrinsic validity, in terms of the kind of conditioning she has experienced in life.

- Help him discover that the more guilt, shame and hatred he attaches to his stuttering, the more he will hold back, and the more he will be likely to stutter. Help him explore and share and diminish these loads of negative emotionality.

- Deal with the **here** and **now.** Emphasize the possibilities of the future, not the mistakes of the past. "Where do we go from here? What behavior choices are available? What can I do at this point?" Those are the questions that lead somewhere. Questions or statements like, "If only I hadn't done this," or "I wish this had happened differently," or "I am a failure," or "Why do things always go wrong for me?" tend to lead to nowhere.

- Let the stutterer know that you are interested in more than just the stuttering, that you are interested in her as a person. Get to know and understand her as a person as thoroughly as you can. She is better off if she feels you care about her and her feelings, that you are on her side whether she is a success or a failure in society's eyes, and that your emotional support doesn't have strings and conditions attached to it.

- Be on the lookout for signs that he is trying to pretend more progress than he is actually experiencing, just to please you and retain your support.

- As she reduces her load of shame, guilt, frustration and despair, help her prepare for the probability that progress and eventual recovery from the handicap of stuttering may still leave her with other problems with which she must cope. She may have to modify her view that stuttering has been the only impediment to her success; she may discover other problems, along with newly realized problems.

- Beware of therapy-induced guilt, and at least be able to recognize it even if you can't entirely prevent some guilt development during the course of therapy. With a habit-based problem such as stuttering, it commonly happens that the stutterer finds, after coasting or wallowing in new-found fluency, he experiences an apparent return of the feelings and behaviors he thought he had conquered (Jost's Law of Habits). Unless continually practiced for a time, newly acquired responses drop out faster than older and more long-established response patterns. With relapse comes guilt—but the client can be prepared for the possibility, and can reestablish his improvement by the methods he used during therapy.

- Every client should be encouraged to develop initiative and independence of the therapist, and can learn in time to become her own clinical resource. The therapist can help the stutterer shift from early dependence to later independence.

- Fostering independence is not the same as abandonment, and the stutterer must always feel free to return to the clinician if new problems arise, or if he needs a refresher on dealing with the old ones.

- Since some overlearning of newly acquired feelings and learned behavior patterns is desirable, the stutterer should not be dumped out of therapy the moment he becomes fluent, or more fluent than formerly. Stabilization for a considerable time after initial improvement is usually needed to protect the gains made during the therapy and to continue an abiding interest in the person and what he does with his life after improvement or recovery from the handicap of stuttering.

Chapter 4

counseling parents of children who stutter

Diane G. Hill, M.A.

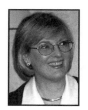

Main goals of counseling parents

Parent counseling should be a key element of any approach to treating children who stutter. It is critical to treatment effectiveness to have significant contact with parents. As discussed in the Stuttering Foundation video *Counseling: Listening to and Talking with Parents of Children who Stutter* (Stuttering Foundation DVD No. 9122), the way parents feel, think and behave contributes to the child's environment and influences treatment progress. Parents know their children and want the best for them. When we as clinicians take the time to listen to parents' concerns and elicit their observations and insights, we validate them and begin to develop a positive relationship.

Building a trusting relationship provides the foundation for successful counseling, education and changes in emotional and behavioral response. The four main goals of counseling parents of children who stutter are to help them: 1) express their feelings, thoughts and beliefs about the problem; 2) make the connection between their emotions and actions, 3) manage their emotions through activities that transform or "bind" free-floating emotions into positive actions, and 4) provide educational information about the problem of stuttering and how they can make changes to support the treatment process. The overarching end goal of counseling is to assist parents in coming to accept the problem and their feelings about the problem and to cope positively in dealing with their child and his stuttering problem.

The Clinician-Parent Partnership

What does it take to build a trusting relationship with parents of a child who stutters? First, it takes time. Parents respond positively when they feel professionals are sincere in their efforts to listen to them. It is important to realize that both building a relationship and beginning the treatment process start with the first contact we have with parents.

During the first contact with a parent, usually via telephone, I try to make sure that I have the time, at least 20 minutes, to listen to them tell their story. I usually begin with an **open-ended question** such as "What is concerning you about your child?" At this stage I want to **listen actively** and affirm the parent's sharing of feelings, thoughts and worries. It is important not to jump too quickly to giving advice but first to gain as much understanding of the problem as possible. I might say, "It sounds as though you are worried that your child is developing a significant stuttering problem. How can I be of help?" I then tailor the educational information in response to the questions parents ask. Information will be more actively used if it relates to what the parents say they need to know. Whether the parents are just seeking information or they wish to schedule a diagnostic assessment, the way the clinician converses with them in an unhurried, non-judgmental, client-centered, supportive manner will encourage them to move forward on the journey of learning about and managing their child's stuttering problem. It will set the tone for further interactions. Whatever the course of action recommended, I want to reinforce the notion that the parent is the expert on the child and their participation is a much-needed and valued part of a diagnostic or treatment process.

A second step in building trust, as discussed by Luterman (2001), requires the clinician to demonstrate reliability and credibility. To demonstrate reliability, I make sure to follow through, respond in a timely manner and behave consistently with parents. To establish credibility, I need to show that I am knowledgeable. The information I provide must be sound, based on research, and widely accepted by experts in the field of stuttering. Although there are many benefits to living in the information age with a great deal of information available on the Internet, parents often become confused when they receive conflicting information. I need to help parents reduce this confusion. On the other hand, I need to be open with parents if I do not have knowledge or experience with specific issues. We will not lose credibility if we are honest about our expertise, work to gain needed knowledge and experience or refer to other professionals who are more specialized.

The third step in building a relationship with parents is to value their opinions. If parents feel their ideas are valued, they are then able to receive needed information about treatment and participate actively. One mother shared with me that "knowledge is power." She had come from another treatment center and was not invited to observe or trained to carry out home practice. She was in the dark and felt confused and unsure what was expected from her. Maintaining open communication is crucial for progress and problem solving to continue

The Initial Contact:
Encouraging Open Communication

As Hugo Gregory discussed in Chapter One, clinicians' attitudes about themselves and the client influence the way they communicate and respond. It is important to be open to the unique situation and needs of each family we work with. Furthermore, it is essential not to prejudge what factors within the child or the environment may be contributing to the child's stuttering problem. Thus we want to begin by making the parents the focal point of our initial interaction. We want them to feel comfortable sharing what they feel, think and believe about their child's stuttering problem. The way we pose questions, listen actively, as described by Carl Rogers (1951), and respond (Luterman, 2001; Shipley, 1992) will make a significant difference. Always beginning with **open-ended questions** (i.e., a question to which parents can respond in any number of ways) will encourage parents to express what is concerning them the most. For example, I might say "Tell me as much as you can about how you feel about Julie's stuttering." Remember the first goal of counseling is to help parents express their feelings, thoughts and beliefs. So as we listen and respond to the parents' answer we will want to be ready to respond with follow-up with more **closed questions** (i.e. questions parents respond to specifically). For example, I might say "How long has Julie been stuttering?" or a **continuing remark** such as "I see. It must be difficult for you to feel so anxious." Another way to help parents share and probe for emotional content is to **paraphrase or restate the parent's message,** for example, "So you feel that you caused Julie's stuttering problem because you returned to work and weren't able to spend as much quality time with her?" I want to allow time for parents to process questions and respond fully. A calm, unhurried, empathetic demeanor will help parents feel comfortable sharing more fully.

When human beings cannot communicate without struggle people close to them experience varying degrees of emotional distress. Emotions shared by parents of children with communication disorders include feelings of inadequacy, vulnerability and confusion as well as grief, anger, and guilt. As parents share their feelings, I want to be accepting by listening and valuing what the parents have to say. We use **affirmation** with indications that we hear them, such as non-verbal encouragements like a nod or an "uh huh." I might also respond with **affect responses** such as, "It must hurt you to think that others might not accept your child because he stutters." In these ways, I am modeling acceptance of the feelings parents share. Helping parents express their feelings is the first step toward acceptance and change.

In addition to encouraging parents to "tell their story," I want to respond appropriately to questions they have. However, it is important to maintain **active listening** to demonstrate my belief that the parents are the experts when it comes to knowing their child and how to best help him. So for example, if a parent says, "Why does Jack stutter more on weekends?" rather than discussing possible reasons such as reduced structure and routine during weekends, we might want to use a **counter question** asking for the parent's own ideas, for example, "What do you think might contribute?"

Many other questions parents ask require factual responses: "Will my child grow out of stuttering?", "Is stuttering a psychological problem?" or "How early should I start treatment?" The educational information I give will help reduce confusion and the sense of vulnerability parents may have developed because of lack of information or misinformation. Here the responses the clinician gives are **content responses,** providing sound educational information. I always recommend that the parents obtain published information pertinent to the age of their child to reinforce the information given, to provide more detailed information, and to serve as a reference for the parents over time. Some of the resources available, published by the Stuttering Foundation, include books *Stuttering and Your Child: Questions and Answers, If Your Child Stutters: A Guide for Parents,* and the DVD *Stuttering and Your Child: Help for Parents.*

At the conclusion of this initial contact, I want to assist parents in determining a course of action. First, some general suggestions should be given about how parents can help their preschool or school age child by listening and responding in an attentive, supportive manner, and observing the environment to determine how communicative stress might be reduced.

Second, parents should be assured that by working together with their child and a clinician who is knowledgeable about stuttering problems, progress can be made in improving fluency, overall communication and attitudes about communication.

Third, the parents and I should determine what type of evaluation or treatment seems best for their child. I cannot state too strongly my bias toward recommending an evaluation first to gain as complete an understanding as possible of the factors involved before making specific recommendations for treatment.

Finally I talk with the parents about how they might prepare their child for meeting the clinician. It is important for clinicians and parents to match their explanations about stuttering and what they are planning to do to help as closely as possible to the child's understanding and expectations. Here I help parents begin to feel more comfortable talking about talking and talking about stuttering. I give them permission to talk about something they may have been afraid to mention. For the young preschool child they might comment "That was a little hard to say. That's o.k. You're still learning to talk." Or for the older child parents might say, "Sometimes you repeat sounds or hold on to sounds. That's called stuttering. We're going to learn more about it with you."

Involving Parents in the Treatment Process

As the diagnostic process ends, I want to spend time with parents providing feedback about our findings. As David Luterman (2001) advises, we will probably be more effective if we talk about what the parents want to know rather than if we run through a long list of test findings. I want to give parents time to respond as we discuss my understanding of their child's stuttering problem. Parents, particularly mothers, may share a sense of guilt that they caused the problem, didn't seek help early enough, or did not monitor treatment more closely. I want to help parents recognize that they have taken action because of their deep feelings of concern. They have sought help. I want to help parents focus more on the "here and now." Helping parents recognize that what they do now will determine how their child makes progress and will help reduce their anxiety.

Clinicians need to recognize the importance of educating parents about stuttering and the best ways to respond and support change—both their own and their child's. I reassure them, focus them on the present, and bind their emotions by

- providing findings from the evaluation
- educating them about the treatment process
- giving them specific positive things to do

I spend time explaining that working with children to develop fluency skills involves the whole family. Everyone will participate in sessions and learn how to support fluency skill development. Further, time will be spent discussing parents' observations and questions. I teach parents how to identify types of disfluency and comment about them as we observe sessions or view videotape together. I might say such things as "That's an easy word repetition — that's typical disfluency," or "Did you hear the difference in that repetition of the syllable in bu bu bu but?" "There was some tension and he speeded up during the repetition. That's more characteristic of stuttering."

Next, I instruct parents to chart (see example below) several episodes of increased disfluency/stuttering between visits. They are asked to note who the child is speaking to, what message is conveyed, what characterizes the stuttering behavior, the child's awareness of stuttering, how the listener reacts to the stuttering and the message, and identify fluency disrupting influences that may have contributed to the child's stuttering. Some possible child factors are:

- being excited
- gaining listener attention
- expressing complex thoughts

Examples of environmental stress include

- rapidly paced, overlapping conversation
- requests for verbal performance
- exposure to new situations and changes in routine

By paying attention to the interaction between speaker and listener, and noting situational factors that may contribute to fluency breakdown, parents begin to make discoveries about significant child or environmental factors.

Charting of Difficult Speaking Situations

Person	Message	Child's Awareness of Difficulty	Type of Disfluency	Listener Reaction	Child's Reaction	Pressures of the Situation
Older friend, Mike	Mike asked Brad to play with him but he was getting ready for school	He was tense, but not aware of disfluencies	Repetitions— when he asked Mom if he could play	Mother reassured Brad that he could play after school	Calmed down, more fluent	Excitement, time pressure conflict, wanted to play yet had to go to school

As I discuss the parents' observations, listen to their concerns and answer questions, I am helping them make the connection between their emotions and actions. For example, one parent discovered that she was interrupting her son when he stuttered because it was painful to hear. Another mom realized that she ordered for her daughter in a restaurant because she didn't want her to stutter in front of others. These parents were not accepting of stuttering because it was hurtful or embarrassing to them. *Parents need to express and accept their emotions before they can make changes in their behavior.*

At this stage of counseling, I want to reinforce the parents' insight and accept the feelings they express. I respond with comments such as "It seems as though you've discovered a reason that you interrupt your son. It's painful for you to listen to him stuttering. That's a good insight." As treatment progresses, it will be important to reinforce parents' behavior changes. If changes do not occur, it will be necessary to be more direct, pointing out how changes in interactive style would be beneficial to the child's development of fluency skills and possibly practicing new behaviors with the parents. For example, it may be useful for me to view a videotape of the parents interacting with their child, pointing out to them changes they might make that would be beneficial to treatment.

As parents learn to understand treatment procedures and expectations for them and the child, the clinician is helping them adopt realistic expectations for change. They need to be prepared for the ups and downs in frequency and severity of stuttering that are inherent in the problem. Parents are often devastated when they observe backsliding after a long period of improved fluency. This happens when the habit strength of fluency skills is not yet strong enough to balance the effects of internal or external stresses. For example, a mother in the Stuttering Foundation's video *Counseling: Listening to and Talking with Parents of Children who Stutter* shared her feeling of panic when her daughter began to stutter during a break from treatment during holidays. She acknowledged her realization that the problem was more chronic than she thought initially. There was no quick fix. "It wasn't something you could put a band aid on and take care of it. It was something that was more long term and you really had to be vigilant." When she realized that there were things she could do to help by modeling easy speech, calming down the environment and providing more structure, she learned that she could make a significant difference. She commented, "I felt stronger when I started modeling easy speech and my daughter picked up on the cues immediately. So it wasn't learning for the first time." She had been empowered to be an agent of change and she felt good about it. She was reinforced for playing a key role.

I guide parents in making decisions about how to implement changes to achieve the following goals:

- show unconditional love, acceptance and support for the child;
- spend quality one-on-one time with the child. Seek ways to build their self-esteem, learn about a child's skills and interest and follow their lead;
- model interactive behaviors conducive to fluency development;
- consider the effects of various life events, activities, school placement and scheduling on their child's speech and overall well being. Modify as needed;
- examine expectations for child behaviors and provide consistent discipline and routines;
- promote generalization of fluency skills to the home environment and assume a primary role in montoring and problem-solving as treatment phases out.

During the later stages of treatment, the clinician's role as a coach, guiding the parent in developing skills and problem solving is reduced to that of a consultant to whom the parents report observations, address questions and ask for assistance when needed. Some parents have a difficult time with termination from treatment and earlier-felt emotions may resurface. As another mother on the "counseling video" shared, "I'm worried that it's going to come back... I'm nervous that if we let go completely that it's going to come back." By gradually phasing out of treatment, lessening treatment sessions over a period of months, and then scheduling rechecks, parents and clinicians can determine the stability of fluency and the parents skills in managing residual stuttering on their own. Clinicians need to be open to parents' feelings of fear and worry about the future. At the same time we need to encourage independence by presenting possible future scenarios and discussing with parents how they would manage these situations. I include parents in goal setting, involve them in designing home practice tasks, and rely on them for monitoring and reporting on the status of their child's fluency. During the last phase of treatment, prior to the child's dismissal, I prepare the family, over at least a period of weeks, for the child's dismissal. Both parents and children are encouraged to talk with me about what they liked/didn't like about the experience; what was hard or easy; what they would like to do or learn before ending treatment; and what they would like to have as a remembrance. Of course both the parents and child need to know that they can call or visit me at any time.

Working with the Extended Family

The involvement of all family members, most importantly both parents, will help immensely in gaining a full understanding of a child's stuttering problem and increase the chances that treatment will be successful. As Luterman (2001), Andrews and Andrews (1990), Gregory and Gregory (2002) discuss, one part of a family cannot really be understood apart from others in the family group. Many counselors base treatment on a family system model. The premise of this model is that everyone in a family is affected by the behavior of one member and that in order to change behavior everyone must communicate about and work together to support the change. If the family system does not support the change in behavior, change may not be "allowed" to occur or progress in treatment may be undermined. Focusing on and behaving in a way to maintain the stuttering problem may allow family members to be distracted from more serious problems in the family. We need to be alert to the need to help families identify these problems and refer for professional help beyond our expertise. The more clinicians understand about the roles family members play—the ways they interact, the things they enjoy or don't enjoy doing—the better they can match the type of information provided and specific assignments given.

Counseling Both Parents

It is important for clinicians to listen to and value the unique perspectives, emotions and beliefs that each parent has to share. In diagnostic interviews, feedback sessions, observation of treatment, and parent conferences, we need to work hard to include both parents and to be sure to give them both an opportunity to communicate. Sometimes I have heard parents says "My husband doesn't seem as concerned as I am about Sally's stuttering" or "I find it difficult to explain what's going on in treatment with Sally's grandmother" or "I try hard to model easy speech at home, but my husband finds it hard to support by doing it too." By talking with parents at the same time, I provide a neutral setting for them to express and recognize each other's feelings and beliefs. I share information with both parents and discuss their reactions and questions, clarifying points of view and summarizing what they think and feel. By modeling positive regard for both parents and accepting differing points of view, I encourage ongoing communication. As I guide parents in assuming their important roles during treatment, I encourage each parent to make changes in ways that feel right to them and for each parent to support the other in their efforts.

In the counseling video a father revealed how much stronger "the power of two" parents working together can be. He said "I didn't always see the improvement as much as my wife. Once I started working with her and coming home from work in the evening in a much calmer way, slowing everyone down when they ran up to the door, and working on some things we've learned at the clinic about easy speech, I've noticed it really helps my daughter." This was a powerful conversation. The father was proud of his wife for taking the lead, and she felt supported by his efforts.

In my work at the Northwestern University Speech and Language Clinic, I strongly encouraged both parents to be present for the diagnostic interview and the feedback session. For preschool children, mothers usually attend treatment sessions but I required fathers to attend at least parts of two sessions every two and a half months. I would reschedule sessions if necessary to make it possible for them to participate. For our school-age group, both parents must enroll with their child one evening per week. This makes it possible for them to participate in treatment, attend parent group meetings, and, from first hand experience, develop understanding of the treatment approach and adopt realistic expectations for improvement.

Other Family Members and Caregivers

According to Luterman (2001), grandparents may be an underused resource to families and professionals when it comes to working with children with communication disorders. While grandparents may take longer to recognize a problem, their emotions usually are closely aligned with the parent's. The pain they feel may be increased because of their feelings of hurt for their own child—the parent—and for their grandchild as well. Parents may seek support from their own parents because they want to be parented or they may have ignored the grandparents entreaties to recognize the problem and seek help. Depending on the closeness of the grandparents and the degree to which they are involved in the child's life, it may be important to include them in observing and participating in treatment sessions and spending some time listening to their concerns and encouraging them to share their feelings. I have worked with several sets of grand-parents who were the primary team partners in the treatment process. From this experience, I learned that it is very important to arrange counseling and treatment sessions for both parents and grandparents to be present so that we "stay on the same page," maintain positive regard for all involved, and clarify assign-ments and responsibilities.

Many children live in homes where both parents work. As I counsel families about the treatment process, I tell them that from my experience we see the best results when both parents participate even minimally. I inform them that although I will be the coach, they must "quarterback," determining how the treatment program will be implemented in the home. So scheduling treatment first thing in the morning, at noon time or last thing in the day often might make it possible for one parent to participate at least for a portion of one session each week. When nannies or babysitters bring children to treatment, I want them to participate but I do not want the parents to abdicate their role as the primary team member and decision-maker about changes in the home environment. Communication lines need to remain active to avoid blame for lack of follow-through or progress. Therefore, clinicians need to schedule periodic conferences for all to attend and communicate openly about concerns and assignments.

Parent Group Counseling

Parents of children who stutter often experience feelings of isolation as they try to cope with their feelings and determine how they should respond. Two parents in the counseling video stated that they didn't know anyone else who was experiencing what they were facing. Feeling alone with perceptions, thoughts and feelings can reinforce a sense of guilt. "What is wrong with me? What have I done to cause my child to stutter? I am responsible."

First, participating in a group with other good and caring parents who have had similar thoughts is perhaps the most powerful way to deal with the issue of loneliness. When parents hear others express similar thoughts and mirror their own feelings they begin to realize that they are not alone with their emotions and concerns. "I'm not irrationale; other parents feel as responsible as I do."

Next, the group provides a supportive and accepting environment for parents to share worries and concerns, and see how others have begun to cope positively. This gives parents hope that they too will be able to improve their own situation.

Third, working with parents in a group is efficient and perhaps the most effective way to provide information. Information is not only provided by the leader-clinician but also by the parents themselves. As I lead groups, I am always struck by the fact that the discussion and knowledge imparted is always expanded and pushed further because of the mutual sharing that takes place among the participants. The issues raised provide direction for including content in future meetings that is most pertinent to group members concerns. For example, parents of preschool children may find that child development milestones or principles of discipline would be the most meaningful topics to discuss. However, I take care to keep the focus of these topics on how they relate to dealing with the child's stuttering problem. For example,

I help parents make the link between consistency in discipline and reducing tension and conflict in a way that creates an environment conducive to fluency development. For parents of preschoolers, I provide education (Gregory and Hill, 1989, 1993, 1999; Hill, 2002) about:

- speech, language, and fluency development
- the nature of stuttering
- factors related to persistence of stuttering
- how parents can support fluency development
- interaction of child and environmental factors that may impede or support progress
- involving family members in treatment
- developing home practice programs.

For parents of school-age children, topics may include:

- how stuttering develops and is maintained
- how to talk about stuttering with their child
- how to talk to the child about their feelings and their emotions,
- the treatment process
- communication with the child's teachers
- teasing and bullying
- the role of parents in treatment.

It is important to present the information in a discussion format, always eliciting parents observations, experiences and questions. All group leaders should remain alert to the needs of the group and allow the agenda to change. In my experience no two groups are the same and each group develops its own dynamic interaction. A successful group will begin to lead itself with minimal direction. The group members help select topics of greatest importance and help solve the problems they face. Early in my experience as a clinician, I talked more and kept a tight rein on the agenda. As I gained confidence, I realized that parents benefited most from freely expressing their feelings and concerns as they talked with each other. I often observe parents and children making plans for outings or play dates outside of the clinic. Support systems often develop out of the experience of mutual sharing in the parent group.

In my experience, the best way to work with parents is to involve them in regularly scheduled meetings (Hill, 2002). Whenever possible, I prefer to include four to six parents of preschool children within 18 months of each other in age and school age children within three years of each other in age because many of the concerns raised relate to child development or school issues. Parents are more apt to relate and engage in problem solving together if they face similar issues. Parent group meetings are part of the treatment program and meetings are held weekly for 45 minutes concurrent with one of the two child treatment sessions per week. Parents observe and participate during the second session each week.

The greatest benefit of group meetings occurs early in the treatment process and I normally conduct parent groups for twenty weeks. The opportunity for parents to have group experiences is so important it outweighs the need to make groups homogenous with regard to the child's age. For example it is better to set up monthly meetings of all parents of children who stutter within a school district rather than not to have any parent meetings at all.

Clinicians should learn the necessary leadership skills to successfully manage groups. Effective leaders show their concern by modeling support and showing acceptance, warmth and genuineness. Leaders encourage group participants to be open, take risks and make changes. Other helpful leadership skills include exploring, clarifying, interpreting and providing guidelines for change. For groups to run smoothly and stay focused, leaders also need to set rules, manage group time and encourage each member to assume responsibility. It has been said that if leaders take up less than 25 percent of group time talking, it is usually a successful group. It is important to provide content responses to questions but to always balance these responses with encouraging interactions within the group. Finally, it may be important for the leader to use additional strategies to move the group forward in making some changes. Challenging, confronting, and, on occasion, self-disclosing are used to encourage parents to take initiative and follow-through.

To conclude, the partnership that develops between the clinician, parents, extended family members and caregivers will provide a framework for change. Establishing a trusting relationship, based on caring, listening, affirming and encouraging will support this change. From the beginning stages of treatment to the termination of clinical services, we shift roles as we encourage parents to assume ever greater responsibility for change. It is very important for all members of the team, clinicians as well, to understand that modifying attitudes and changing behaviors is a process that occurs over time, and varies depending on the nature of the problem. I want to encourage parents to value each step of progress and recognize their child's as well as their own achievements in supporting fluency development and improving communication.

Bibliography

Ainsworth, S. and Fraser, J. (2012). *If your child stutters: A guide for parents.* 8th ed. Memphis, TN: Stuttering Foundation of America (pub. 0011).

Andrews, J. and Andrews, M. (1990). *Family based treatment in communication disorders: A systematic approach,* Sandwich, Illinois: Janelle Publications, Inc.

Conture, E. and Fraser, J. (2002). *Stuttering and your child: Questions and answers.* 4th edition. Memphis, TN: Stuttering Foundation of America. (pub. no. 0022, 2010 reprinted).

Gregory, H. and Gregory, C. (1999). Counseling children who stutter and their families. In R. Curlee (Ed.), *Stuttering and related fluency disorders* (pp. 43–64). New York: Thieme.

Gregory, H. and Hill, D. (1999). Stuttering therapy for preschool children. In R. Curlee (Ed.), Stuttering and related fluency disorders (pp. 351–364). New York: Thieme.

Hill, D. (2002). Differential treatment of stuttering in the early stages of development. In H. Gregory (Ed.), *Stuttering therapy: Rationale and procedures.* New York: Allyn and Bacon.

Luterman, D. (2001). *Counseling persons with communication disorders and their families.* 4th ed. Austin, TX: Pro-Ed.

Rogers, C. (1951). *Client centered therapy.* Boston: Houghton Mifflin.

Shipley, K. (1992). *Interviewing and counseling in communication disorders: Principles and disorders.* New York: Merrill, Macmillian Publishing Company.

Chapter **5**

talking with children who stutter

Dean E. Williams, Ph.D.

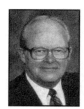 *Editor's Note: Dean Williams established an outstanding national and international reputation as a clinician, researcher, and teacher in the area of stuttering. As a person who stuttered himself, Williams made many significant contributions, one of which was his 1957 essay,* "A Point of View about Stuttering," *in which he defined an objective way to think about stuttering, while also laying the groundwork for his "normal talking" model of fluency therapy. In the "normal talking" model, children who stutter are encouraged to see their stuttering behavior as something they do to interfere with the process of normally fluent speech. In this way, they learn that the same speech production processes, used differently, underlie both their fluent and disfluent speech. From this perspective, children can appreciate that stuttering is not something that "happens to them." Therapy, then, involves helping children to become physically aware of what they do when they talk, both fluently and disfluently, and how to change stuttered speech into speech that is "normally (dis)fluent."*

In this chapter, first published in 1981, Dr. Williams describes a way to talk with children who stutter about their stuttering, a process that he considered integral to the "normal talking" therapy model. Specifically, Williams stated that by talking frankly and openly with children about what they believe stuttering is, why they believe they stutter, and what they think helps them to talk better, clinicians can provide them with the information they need to talk the way they want. As Dr. Williams discusses in the following pages, these

clinician-child conversations should involve an active process of directing children to observe the way they talk, and then helping them to explore their perceptions of these observations.

There is a general agreement among most speech-language clinicians that some form of counseling is appropriate for adolescents and adults who stutter. There is not similar agreement, however, of its appropriateness for children of elementary school age. Often, there is disagreement about what counseling involves and how it can be "adapted" to children. Stated simply, counseling involves talking **with** another person. Of course a clinician **talks with** a child so the confusion must arise over the purpose of talking with them.

...counseling involves talking **with** another person.

The purpose of talking with children who stutter is to discuss with them frankly and openly their beliefs about what they believe is wrong, what they believe helps them talk better, and what their feelings are about talking. Once this is determined, they need information about what talking involves and what they can do constructively in order to talk the way they want to talk. The talking that is done is structured around an active process of directing observations as the children are experiencing the ways they are talking and then helping the children evaluate and re-evaluate their interpretations of those observations. The goal is to help children explore the reality of what they are doing and to introduce and demonstrate the alternatives they have for change. Said in another way, counseling is directed toward assisting children to learn the elements of problem solving with regard to stuttering.

To do this most effectively, clinicians cannot be indirect, cannot be coy and skirt around issues or topics, cannot assume the stereotype "teacher" role of **telling** the children what to learn, cannot talk "down" to them or on the other hand, adopt a "professional" language that is vague at best and scary at worst.

Instead, a clinician should enter each child's language experience world and function from there. Most children will talk common sense with the clinician if the clinician will talk common sense with them.

Beliefs

Children who stutter generally receive much information about stuttering and many instructions of "what to do" or "what not to do" that are confusing and misleading. Before the clinician begins to explain the therapy programs to a child, it is desirable to find out as much as possible about the child's beliefs about what his stuttering is. If this is not done, the child is likely to interpret the clinician's statements and therapy activities from a perspective of distorted and perhaps erroneous beliefs of what is wrong with his speech and what he perceives he has to do to improve. Hence, as clinical activities are presented and the child filters their purposes (as explained) through his own belief system, he is apt **to learn** things that are different from what the clinician intended **to teach.** Even though positive changes in speech are attained in the therapy room, the child's ability to transfer and to maintain them in all speaking situations becomes precarious when such changes are built on a foundation of the shifting sands of confused beliefs.

Talking with the children about what they **believe** is wrong and what they do that they believe helps them talk better can assist the clinician in providing meaningful information about the problem. Also, it assists in explaining the purposes of the proposed therapy program that are meaningful to a child — because they take into account the child's own view of the problem. Children differ in their beliefs as to what is wrong and what is helpful. Clinicians should be aware of this. Such awareness prevents them from falling into a ritualized "sameness" as they begin therapy with different children.

Most children's beliefs about why they have trouble talking (what's wrong) are often fragmentary and vague. Others just shake their heads and say that they don't know. Still others are quite imaginative and specific. Explanations from "words get stopped in my mouth" to "words get hooked in my throat on little fish hooks," deserve thoughtful consideration by a clinician as to their implications for what the children are trying to do as they talk to conquer the problem as they perceive it. Regardless of the reasons given by a child, they deserve and require respectful discussion with the child; not from a perspective of implying that the idea is silly or wrong or unimportant, but from the standpoint of listening, of questioning, of thinking aloud with the child what it means—of sharing with the child his dilemma. **No conclusions need to be drawn at the time.**

If the child seems to be confused or frightened by his uncertainties, the clinician can reflect these or similar feelings by stating something like, "It's confusing isn't' it?" Or "It's kind of scary to not have any idea what's wrong isn't it? You're trying to talk and all of a sudden things just go whambo!" The clinician can terminate the discussion by stating something like, "Look, we'll come back and discuss this some more when we start talking about what you can do to help yourself improve the ways you talk."

The next area of beliefs to be discussed is **what the children have been doing to help themselves talk better.** If they have beliefs about what is wrong, the things they do to help themselves ordinarily grow out of those beliefs of what is wrong. For example, the child who stated that "the words got hooked in his throat on little fish hooks," **pushed hard** in order to "slip the words off the hooks" so he could "get them out." Clinicians should realize that children's beliefs create strong motivations for the ways they behave. If changes are attempted in the ways a person behaves without taking into consideration the motivations which prompt the behavior—even if changes are accomplished—they are apt to be unstable at best unless there are corresponding changes in the motivation for the behavior. This requires, often, an examination of the beliefs that are the guiding force for the motivation.

There are children who have no explainable reasons for what they believe is wrong, but few have no idea of what they can do to "help." Many of these ideas come from what they have been told by others. For example, two of the most common instructions they receive are "relax" and "slow down." The following conversations with children will illustrate the perplexing incongruity the children face between what they try to do to help, what they do, and their explanations for it.

First child in a conversation with the clinician.

SLP: **"So, you're talking along and all of a sudden you stutter. Why do you suppose it happens right there?"**

C: "Oh, I stutter when I talk too fast."

SLP: **"You do? How did you find that out?"**

C: "Well, when I stutter, they tell me to slow down."

SLP: **"Mmm-hmm, do they even tell you to slow down when you don't stutter?"**

C: "No."

SLP: **"Why do you suppose they don't?"**

C: "I guess it's because I must be talking slower."

SLP: **"Oh, I see. Well, what do you do to help yourself when you talk?"**

C: "I try to slow down so I won't stutter."

SLP: **"Does that help?"**

C: "Some of the time."

SLP: **"Some of the time?"**

C: "Yeah. You see, I don't stutter all the time."

Second child in a conversation with the clinician:

SLP: **"You say you stutter some. What do you do to help at those times?"**

C: "I try to relax."

SLP: **"Oh, why do you do that—are you real tense?"**

C: "I don't know—they tell me to relax so I won't stutter."

SLP: **"Does it help?"**

C: "Yeah."

SLP: **"All of the time?"**

C: "Yeah, except when I stutter."

SLP: **"Mm-hmm. What do you do then?"**

C: "I just stutter."

SLP: **"And then what do you do?"**

C: "I just don't talk for a while."

SLP: **"You don't talk for a while, I see. Don't you feel like talking, or what?"**

C: "I feel kinda bad. I don't want to talk until I feel better."

Again, as with the earlier discussion, **there is no need for the clinician to confront and resolve the child's beliefs at the time.** The clinician, again, can reflect the child's feelings and possible confusion.

The example of the second child illustrates also how these ways of talking with a child open the door to discussing the child's feelings about stuttering and about himself. For younger children, the feelings are predominately ones of feeling "bad" or "sad." The overriding emotion is one of frustration. Strong embarrassment surfaces with many as they get older. The things they do to help are inconsistently helpful (according to their perceptions) or lead to more difficulty. An example of the latter is the child who said he helped by just pushing the word out. When asked what he did when that didn't help, he replied, "I push harder." They become frustrated because they are doing the only things they know to help themselves—and these things are not too helpful. This leads to doubts about their ability to cope. They are experiencing conflicts about what to do. Things are not working the way they intended. They are developing feelings of helplessness. This is scary to them.

What's Going On?

When a clinician begins to share the particular view that the children have about what is wrong and what they can do to help themselves talk better, it should become obvious that the children need constructive information about what's going on. Stuttering appears to them to be very mysterious. They are confused by it. They are likely to feel that they are "defective" or that something is horribly "wrong with them." They can begin to feel that they are "dumb" or "incompetent" because they cannot overcome the "thing" by gritting their teeth and trying harder. After all, most adults seem to know how they can stop doing it. The children are told, for example, that if they would only "slow down" or "relax" or "think of what they are going to say," they wouldn't do it. It sounds so easy. Yet when they try it, they fail. There appears to be little, if any, relationship between what they do to help and the result of what they do. The trouble must be with **them.**

The clinician has a responsibility to each child to help him learn "what is going on"—what accounts for this disparity between what the child is trying to accomplish and the result. Or, said in a more constructive way, the clinician should help the child learn the relationship between what the child is doing to help and what he is doing to interfere with his speaking. Moreover, it should be done in ways that the child can understand. The word "understand" is used not to refer to a relatively abstract intellectual understanding, but to one based on the child's own world of experiences. He must be able to relate this "understanding" to his everyday activities.

Too often, clinicians begin by talking and philosophizing about stuttering by attempting to define it. This results in an explanation that includes the statement, "There are many different reasons given for stuttering. No one knows, for sure what causes it, but we'll do what we can to help you."

This type of explanation easily can convey to the child that the clinician is as confused as he is, but something will be "tried." The compulsion that we have in our profession to discover "the cause" spills over into our clinical procedures. The child is not interested in the confusion among stuttering theoreticians. He wants to know "what is going on" when he begins to talk and what he can do about it. This is reasonable. Instead of attempting to define stuttering, we need to **explain** to the child "what's going on" in a way 1) that reassures him that something terrible is not wrong with **him** and 2) conveys a positive direction involving constructive learning experiences.

My own personal preference is to explain it in terms of learning. The child is in the midst of the experiences of learning. He is learning at school, he is learning to get along with friends, he is learning, learning, learning. He knows what it means. Moreover, there is little doubt that learning is **normal**. At the same time, it can be explained in ways that do not violate most responsible theories about the development of the stuttering problem. An example of the essentials of such an explanation follows:

Stuttering is a confusing thing to most boys and girls. It's tough to know what one can do about it. It seems at times it's almost like a "burp." You can feel it coming and, whoops, you burp! About the only thing you can do is press your lips tightly together so it won't sound too loud — or put your hand over your mouth so people won't notice it too much. Although stuttering may seem to be something like that, it really isn't. Stuttering is something you began to do when you were learning to talk. We all have to learn to talk — just like we have to learn to read or do arithmetic. When we learn, we make mistakes. This is a normal part of learning anything. It's true with learning to talk. Examples are demonstrated of different types of disfluencies which make up the mistakes of talking. It's no different from learning arithmetic. Some children make more mistakes than others when they learn arithmetic. Some make fewer. The same is true with reading — or with talking. But regardless, as we practice and learn, we get so we can do arithmetic, or read, or talk OK.

You probably made more mistakes when you were learning to talk than some of the other children did. You didn't want to make so many so you began to fight them. The harder you fought, the more mistakes you made. It's kind of like learning to catch a ball. (Or any other similar type of behavior.) If you try hard to "not drop the ball" — or tense up and "pounce" at it so you won't goof, you drop it more often. This is the way it is when you do what we call "stuttering." You fight to say it right. When you fight, you tense, you may pounce (quick increase in velocity of movement). Or you may generally "hold back." When you do this you tense, maybe hold your breath and get set to "fight any mistakes you may make." This is a very normal reaction — a normal way to fight mistakes. You're OK. There is nothing inside you — in your mouth or throat or stomach that stops a word. You learn to fight your speech. You can learn to talk smoothly.

The above explanation is **not presented in a monologue.** One includes the child in the discussion by asking if he understands, by asking for other examples, etc. Finally the clinician models different types of disfluencies, then asks the child to do them. Then the clinician models fighting them in different ways and asks the child to do the same. **This aspect may take several therapy sessions.** The child must experience them, explore them, puzzle over them as the clinician and the child discover what he's doing. This then leads into comparing them with what he does during any "real" instances of stuttering. He needs to explore all the facets of the similarities and differences between the "fighting" he does in specified ways and the occurrence of a "real" stutter. The clinician needs to talk with him and examine them too. It's a period of learning, of discovery, of realization that he is doing these things. This is the foundation upon which the task of establishing congruence between intent and resulting behavior is learned.

The next necessary learning experience is to discover that as he changes the ways he "fights," he changes the result—or, the characteristics of the stutter. He should tense up more, then less. He should speed up the velocity of movement, then decrease it, etc. He should talk and not fight so hard when he "stutters." The clinician should be involved by modeling the changes then asking the child to do the same thing. This establishes the foundation for **change.** It involves learning that the reality of changes is dependent on what the child **does.** This opens the door for improved self esteem, for the development of taking responsibility. The child can learn that **he** has something to do with what he does—and that what he does determines what "happens" when he talks.

The purposes of the activities described above should not be confused with those of "desensitizing to stuttering," or with those of "accepting one's stuttering." These are not designed to show the child that he should talk that way out in social situations. They are not therapy techniques aimed at the immediate production of fluency. **They are structured experiences designed in order to guide the observations the child is making.** As he makes them, his perceptions and evaluations can be discussed with him. Different interpretations can be suggested by the clinician and then immediately tested. They can be **a most effective method**

of counseling with children regardless of the therapy procedures employed by the clinician to improve fluency. It requires the child to discuss and evaluate his experiences in the reality of the present instead of from the unreality of his remembrances of the past.

The experiences and discussion described above will ordinarily bring to the surface the child's sensations of emotion. These can be shared and discussed openly. The clinician can lead such discussions in the direction of helping the child learn that attending to and changing one's behavior is dependent on what the child **does** and is not dependent on reducing or eliminating one's emotions. He can learn that he can change the way he does things in the presence of emotion. This is one of the most effective ways for a child to cease depending on his "feelings" to tell him how he will talk. By so doing, the way he "feels" becomes less important and what he does becomes more important during the process of talking. Hence, his **awareness** of "feelings" diminishes.

What Do We Do to Talk?

The question of "What do we need to do to talk?" naturally follows from — or blends into — the above discussion. For the clinician a more meaningful question is, "What does the child have to do to learn correspondence between what he intends to do and what he does?" Too often clinicians attempt to answer the question by imposing on the child a special speech pattern (either of fluency or of stuttering) in order, hopefully, to heal his wounded speech. This approach, it seems, reflects the clinician's limited perspective as much, or more, than it does the child's abilities or inabilities. Such an approach takes advantage, apparently without recognizing it, of the child's beautiful ability to cope and to adapt to a wide variety of ways of talking. Clinicians differ in what they preach and teach. Some extol movement, others air flow or relaxation, or slow movement, or smooth stuttering, or smooth transitions, etc., all with varying degrees of success. The wonderment of it all is that the poor child is able to cope with any or all of these cross-stitched sutures and still talk.

In order for the child to learn to be responsible for the ways he talks, it is important for **him** to problem-solve about what he does that helps him talk and what he does that doesn't help—in fact, what interferes with talking the way he intends. From his exploration of the behavior used to fight mistakes, he is aware that such things as tensing too much, holding his breath, etc., make talking difficult or impossible. It's time to learn what we do when we talk. This involves providing information about what the process of talking involves. "Providing information" does not include teaching him on an intellectual level the technicalities of speech production. It involves **explaining, demonstrating, experiencing** on a doing level the process of blending air, sound, movement, timing, tensing into the production of what we call words, phrases and sentences. Here the clinician can move into each child's beliefs of what he thought was wrong and what he did to help (discussed earlier) into the reality testing arena for accuracy testing of his beliefs.

child to test and discover for himself. Don't just **tell** him to "know it." If you do so, the child may know but he won't know it in an operational-**doing** way. learn by experiencing that what we call a word is by a movement sequence of tongue, jaw and air or sound. Words don't come out of the throat needs to learn by experiencing the way we begin ation of movement with sound or air, the proper amount of tensing necessary, etc. This explanation cannot be done effectively at the level of the words. The clinician leaves the level of words and relies on experiencing and doing—punctuated by words only to direct the observations that are to be more meaningfully experienced.

By experiencing the things necessary to do to talk the way he intends, it becomes more meaningful to contrast these to different things he can do to interfere with the desired process. He can learn the relationship between tensing and increased velocity of movement, between restricting air and the production of sound, etc.

In summary, he learns what we do to facilitate talking and what we do to interfere with it. Furthermore, he learns that stuttering is not something that erupts out of his mouth but, instead, consists of things he does to interfere with talking all along the vocal pathway. In addition, he learns that he **can** change what he is doing **as** he is talking so that it more nearly conforms to what he intends to do. By the continuous attending to the reality of what he is doing and knowing by experience what will help and what will hinder, he has the **time** to change in the ways he desires. This results in his learning that he has a choice. He is free to act in accordance with his choice. This is the goal of obtaining congruence between what a person intends and the way he behaves.

The intent of this approach to counseling through experience is to ensure in so far as is possible that the child can participate in a program to improve his fluency in a positive, matter-of-fact way. The counseling becomes an integral part of how the clinician helps the child to improve his speech. The child should possess the basic orientation that talking smoothly involves an active doing process to be learned—with the acceptance of the mistakes that accompany any learning.

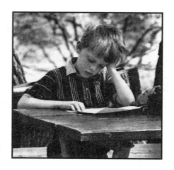

Chapter 6

the severe
young stutterer

Charles Van Riper, Ph.D.

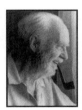 *Editor's Note: Charles Van Riper was a charismatic clinician, teacher, and writer who stuttered severely from his preschool years until his late twenties. He experimented with many ways to improve his own speech and, in the process, developed a therapy that benefited many generations of people who stutter. Dr. Van Riper helped clients confront, explore, and accept their stuttering, thereby reducing the emotions that make stuttering so hard to modify. He then taught clients to stutter in an easier way—free of the abnormal struggle, escape, and avoidance behaviors that evoke listener penalties and interfere with communication.*

Much of Dr. Van Riper's clinical work was done with adults, but in this chapter he describes procedures that clinicians can use to reduce negative emotions in severely stuttering children. Here, he introduces techniques of nonverbal counseling that can help the child express unpleasant feelings about stuttering through gestures and drawings, experience the clinician's acceptance of these feelings, and eventually verbalize them.

In a long career some of the toughest problems that I have encountered have been those presented by very severe young stutterers, especially those who seem chock full of frustration, fear, shame or other unpleasant feelings. These children hurt badly and they show it. Because they find it hard to talk, it is difficult to establish a good clinical relationship. To them, communication is a very painful experience to be undertaken only when absolutely necessary. Often hostile or withdrawn, these children are very difficult to help until some of that bottled up emotion is vented.

These children hurt badly and they show it.

My early attempts to provide some emotional release for these young severe stutterers were the traditional ones: play therapy, simplified verbal counseling, psychodrama, free-smearing techniques and the like. I was not at all impressed with the results I got. While these procedures did enable the children to act out a lot of their conflicts with their parents, siblings or playmates, they did not focus at all on the feelings engendered by the stuttering itself. They could beat up inflated Bozo the Clown enthusiastically but that didn't seem to help them respond to their blockings with any less frustration or struggle. To me, these young stutterers seemed to need some immediate release, some instantaneous way of expressing the feelings that boiled up in them at the moment of stuttering. At first I thought that I could verbalize for them, trying to put into simple words what I thought they were feeling, but it soon became evident that this was not doing the job that needed to be done. The children, shortly after having a very severe moment of stuttering, seemed to be too full of emotion even to hear what I was saying. Moreover, I was doing too much talking and they were doing little or none. Some other way had to be found to help these young severe stutterers ventilate and discharge the unpleasant feelings that arose when they stuttered.

After considerable exploration, I developed some essentially nonverbal techniques that eventually led to the children's being able to share their feelings with me. And then I found not only a marked though temporary increase in fluency but also a willingness or capability for modifying their stuttering behaviors, behaviors that earlier had been very resistant to change.

The essence of this approach requires the clinician to mirror **nonverbally** first the overt stuttering behaviors and then the unpleasant feelings that the child experiences when he stutters. Verbal mirroring, usually termed reflecting, has long been used in psychotherapy, the clinician attempting to verbalize in his own words the feelings being expressed by the client, or which underlie what the latter is telling him. With normal speakers, if the therapist's reflection is inaccurate, the client will verbally reject the interpretation; but many stutterers, and especially the younger severe ones, find this contradicting difficult to do. Therefore, misunderstandings arise that threaten the relationship. Nonverbal mirroring avoids this hazard to some extent since the clinician's symbolic behavior can be interpreted by the child in various ways. Thus he tends to read into it the interpretation most consonant with his actual feelings.

The targets of this nonverbal mirroring are the same ones that have always been viewed as essential: to reduce and help the stutterers cope with their feelings of helplessness, frustration, anger, fear and shame. Improvement in fluency almost always seems to result when these unpleasant responses are weakened, and when they are decreased, both the child and his clinician find the other work of therapy much easier.

... reduce their feelings of helplessness, frustration, anger, fear and shame.

Before we go on to describe the actual procedure of nonverbal mirroring, we should make clear that although the emphasis is upon nonverbal interactions between the clinician and the child, this does not mean that the sessions are completely silent. While the clinician rarely asks a question or insists upon a reply, some brief commentary often occurs; and it is always necessary to do some talking to structure the therapeutic tasks.

We have always begun our therapy with any person who stutters by first exploring together the problem he presents. With a child, we might begin by saying, "I'm going to help you be able to talk more easily but I've got to learn first exactly what happens when you stutter and I guess you'll have to teach me. The next time you have some trouble saying a word, you'll see me having it too. I'm not mocking you; I'm trying to understand what happens."

Then when the child does stutter noticeably we (occasionally) stutter right along with him, trying to duplicate what he is doing. Early in the sessions, we do this on the milder blockings and in pantomime only; but later we will mirror the hard ones too, and aloud. Often we may insert a bit of commentary like this: "No, I didn't do it quite right that time. Forgot to squeeze my lips as tightly as you did. Let me try it again." The major work of the first sessions consists of this mirroring and brief commentary. Sometimes we do it simultaneously with the child; at other times, we echo the stuttering behavior.

Now let us examine the impact of this simple mirroring in terms of its psychodynamics. The child's first reaction is that of surprise; the second, that of suspicion. These soon dissipate as the clinician shows his earnestness and his genuine interest in the stuttering being exhibited. The next reaction is one of relief. The child realizes that here is one adult who is not repelled or appalled by his stuttering. Here in one grown-up who is willing to put into his own mouth the dirty stuff that everyone else rejects or penalizes. And he doesn't seem at all upset or ashamed when he stutters. He's curious about it; he's not afraid to stutter. When these reactions occur, the child no longer feels so terribly alone and helpless. His burden, being shared, is thereby lessened. Perhaps here he has one grown-up he can trust.

In the next phase of this approach the concentration is not primarily on the stuttering behaviors being exhibited but on the feelings that exist concurrently. The clinician introduces this new interaction by saying something like this: "I think I've now pretty well learned what you do when you stutter, and maybe you have too. Now let's see if I can understand how you feel at the time you stutter or just before or afterwards. I'll try to act out what I think your feeling is and if I'm wrong, let me know."

Since the symbolic mirroring of feelings occurs spontaneously and in a specific context, it is difficult to describe it here in print. I know that often I have locked my fingers together and vainly tried to pull them apart when I felt that the child was feeling very frustrated at the moment of hard blocking. There were times when I drooped bodily or whimpered when I thought he was feeling helpless. I have banged the walls and the table if he seemed hostile. There were instances when I covered my face as a gesture of shame, others when I assumed the mask of fear. Often, of course, I failed to mirror the actual feelings, having misinterpreted them, but when that occurred, the child usually corrected me. Once, for example, after a young stutterer had experienced a very long, compulsive series of repetitions that seemed to last interminably, I felt that he must have been terribly frustrated so I banged my fist into the other hand and clenched it hard. "No," said the boy, "It's like this!" and he slapped himself repeatedly in the mouth and kept doing so until I mirrored him, only harder. A great smile came over his countenance. Finally, I had understood.

Often, following one of these symbolic mirrorings, the child will even put his feelings into words. "No, I'm not feeling sad. I'm feeling dirty. Make me an ugly face!" My histrionic ability leaves much to be desired. I'm not much of an actor. But somehow my deficiencies in this regard didn't seem to matter much, perhaps because the child always knew I was really trying to understand how he was feeling and, moreover, was accepting those feelings as being justified and natural. It was enough that for once he could experience those feelings without penalty or self-derogation. Again he learns that he is not alone, and again he feels the great relief that comes when unpleasant feelings are shared with someone he can trust, a relief that results in more fluency.

Another procedure that I have used repeatedly involves projective drawings of the feelings evoked by stuttering. Both of us have a session in which we draw pictures representing anger, fear, helplessness and so forth. Always the child draws something that he calls the "I am mad" or "I'm scared" face and one that shows a face scribbled all over, the "ugly" face for shame. But there are others too: one with a sad expression and tears, another with no mouth at all. One that I remember vividly was just a circle with two huge eyes in it. The child called it his "They're always looking at me" face, and it seemed to represent shame or embarrassment. One picture showed a baby sucking a bottle and the child used it to represent feeling little or helpless.

Sometimes a child will just scribble at random all over the card and will hold it up after a moment of stuttering to show that he doesn't really know how he feels except that he's all mixed up. After we have decided on the cards we want to use, I make a copy of them. Then when the child stutters, we both select the card that we think represents most closely his feelings at that moment and hold it up at the same time to see if we pick the same one. This procedure always stimulates verbalization of the feelings by the child if there are discrepancies. He feels impelled to explain why he chose that card and in the process often reveals many of the rejections and penalties he has received at home or at school. For example, after a long laryngeal blocking in which he struggled vainly to produce a voice on a vowel word, one boy held up the card showing a face without a mouth and then let out one of the best primal screams I've ever heard. Then he said, "Maybe I ought to always yell like that when I get stuck. Like my Dad does at me!" These projective drawings of feelings related to stuttering moments are excellent pump primers.

Any clinician can devise other methods for helping young stutterers express in one way or another the feelings that trouble them. The important point in this little article is that clinicians should recognize the need for such venting in a permissive, caring situation and do something about it.

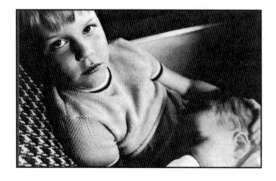

counseling school-age children in group therapy

Barry Guitar, Ph.D., and Julie Reville, M.S.

The Purposes of Group Therapy

We have included a chapter on group therapy for children who stutter in a book about counseling because members of the group are, in effect, counselors for each other. For example, when children share their experiences and their feelings about stuttering, all the members of the group feel supported and understood. In the safety of a situation where everyone else stutters, children feel free to be themselves, to talk despite their stuttering, and to say "Hey, that happened to me, too!" or "That's just how it makes me feel." Our role in a children's group is to plan and guide activities that children enjoy and that give them a chance to talk about their stuttering and learn that it is not so bad after all. Many of the children we work with are also receiving individual therapy. A group gives them a place to practice and improve their skills by watching and listening to each other.

In our clinic a parent group accompanies a children's group, and in this situation, parents are also counselors for each other, providing support, sharing feelings, and helping each other feel supported and understood. When the two groups meet together, parents and children talk to each other, share their feelings, and establish mutual support that continues after the group meetings are over.

School-age children who stutter often feel alone with their stuttering. They are typically the only students in their class who stutter, maybe even the only ones in their school. Family members and the children themselves are rarely comfortable discussing stuttering at home. These circumstances conspire to make the feeling of isolation one of the hallmarks of stuttering in school-age children (Bloodstein, 1995; Guitar, 1998; Van Riper, 1982).

In addition to feeling alone, these children are often saddled with self-conscious feelings—especially those of embarrassment, shame, and guilt. These emotions develop in the late preschool years when children become cognitively mature enough to compare themselves with others. At this age, they know if they have failed to meet the standards around them—in this case, the standards of fluency (Lewis and Haviland-Jones, 2000). Like many negative feelings, embarrassment, guilt, and especially shame increase if they remain hidden away.

In our experience, these children's sense of isolation can be significantly reduced by group therapy. Moreover, such a group can be a place where sharing and discussion bring feelings into the open where they can be dissipated and even transformed into positive feelings like pride.

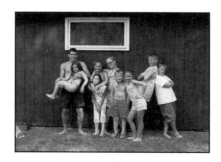

The Structure of Group Therapy

The group therapy format we use has been successful in addressing the feelings of children and parents, as well as improving the communication between them. It is suited to settings where two clinicians are available, one for the parents' group and one for the children's group. Toward the end of this chapter we'll also discuss how a children's group can be run in a school setting with one clinician.

Our approach is to have a clinician meet with a group of children for about an hour while the second clinician meets with their parents during this same hour. Then the parents and their clinician move to the room where the children and their clinician are meeting and a joint meeting continues for about a half-hour. These times should remain flexible because sometimes the parents or the children become deeply immersed in an important issue that needs to be brought to some point of resolution before discontinuing and moving to the combined group. Typically, it's the parent group that occasionally continues a little beyond the hour and may be late in joining the children's group. Sometimes, when we've planned an important activity for the combined group, like making phone calls together, we'll shorten the times the separate groups meet so that there's plenty of time for the combined activity.

We've found that the companionship of eating is an important activity in both groups. In the parent group, we have coffee and tea, as well as a pitcher of ice water on the table. We also have a plate of snacks, like cookies or banana bread. In the children's group, we've learned to delay the snacks until the end of the meeting; otherwise the children are distracted from active participation in the group. We make sure to have parent approval for any food item in treatment.

Our children's group meets in a large room with a circle of chairs — enough for both the children and their parents. We also have a small circular table in the middle of the room for games, pictures, and the end-of-meeting snacks. We've found it important to have something to write on, such as a flip-chart to list the activities we'll have and to brainstorm ideas. For example, in one group the children listed the ways they would like their parents to respond to their stuttering. We also like to have a speaker-telephone in the room. Paper cups are good for collecting tokens and M&M's, used to reinforce such things as sharing feelings and voluntary stuttering. A portable video camera is handy for filming field trips to the mall or the library. We often videotape the group in action and watch the videos in the next session, so a TV monitor is essential.

We've learned that it's important to group the children by similar ages (Conture, 2001). When we first began our group therapy, we had a group of children ages 7 to 15. We discovered, however, that the older children soon lost interest in the activities we designed for the younger children and even sooner lost patience with their misbehavior. Now, depending on the ages we have, we group children more narrowly by age. For example, we may group children from ages 6 to 8, 9 to 11, 12 to 14 and 15 to 18. Sometimes we invite older children who have made progress with their fluency to mentor younger ones. These older children develop self-confidence from this role, and the younger ones look up to them and profit from their example. In addition to mentoring within a group, we sometimes invite teenagers and young adults to visit the younger group and share their experiences with stuttering. This can provide a powerful model for the younger ones.

The Flow of Therapy

First Meeting of the Children's Group. In the first meeting of the children's group, the focus is on getting to know one another and establishing rules for the group. Any "ice-breaker" can be employed to start the group off. One game we've used is to make a grid on the flip-chart in which each row is a different question, marked with the color of an M&M. Questions are designed to help the kids learn about each other. Examples are "What is Your Name?", "Where Do You Live?", "What is Something You Like to Do?" Then a handful of M&M's are given to each child and, one-by-one, each child answers the question and then eats an M&M corresponding to the question's color. The pleasure of eating M&M's counteracts some of the fear associated with talking (and stuttering) in the group. During this activity, there is usually some interrupting, yelling, teasing, or other undesirable behavior. These outbursts then provide an opportunity for the clinician to lead a discussion of what behaviors the group would like to adopt.

Examples are "Let someone talk without interrupting," "Be a good listener," and "Show respect for each other."

First Meeting of the Parents' Group. When the parents first meet, we ask them to introduce themselves and tell a little about their child. To get them started, we let them know it's their group and encourage them to talk about whatever they want. We make ourselves available as a resource to answer their questions about stuttering. From here, the discussion can go in any direction. It takes some experience, some skill, and some courage on our part to be silent and let the group members lead. It's very important to let the group know that we, as the group leaders, have no agenda. We let the group determine its direction (Luterman, 2001).

The most important function of the group is to create a setting in which parents can explore their feelings and thoughts about their child and stuttering, to express those emotions in an accepting environment, and to come to terms with them. For this to happen, the group must become a safe place for parents to share their feelings. This is facilitated if the group creates its own "norms" or rules, for example, that no one has to talk and that group discussions will remain entirely confidential.

Although each parent will have his or her own unique feelings and experiences, many will be common. These may include feelings of isolation and helplessness. Often their child is the only one they know who stutters. Parents may have memories from their own school days of a classmate who stuttered and was teased, rejected, or ignored. Some parents may urgently want their child to receive therapy, but the child may not want therapy. Parents may feel sad because their child stutters. Becoming aware of these feelings and learning that others also feel sad will help them grieve the loss of their dream for a "perfect child." As they relate these feelings in the group, parents support each other and bond as a group. This group support may make it possible for parents to gain more acceptance of themselves and their child.

As parents share their thoughts and their feelings, we comment on both the content and the emotion expressed. This is more than just reflecting what a parent said. We listen for the underlying emotions and comment on them in such a way that parents may recognize feelings and assumptions of which they were previously unaware. Our major role is to be non-judgmental and accepting, and to demonstrate a deep desire to understand parents' experience[1].

First Meeting of the Children and Parents Together. We begin the first combined meeting by stressing that it's important to go ahead and talk whether you stutter or not, stuttering is not something bad, is not anyone's fault, and that talking is cool. Once this open atmosphere is established, we give our names and tell something about ourselves, then have parents tell their names and who their child is. When their turn comes, the children can introduce themselves so that all the parents have an idea of who all the children are.

We have a clear idea beforehand of what the two groups hope to accomplish when they come together. In some instances, the children might plan an activity they want to do with their parents. As they become more familiar with the routine, it is crucial that the children take an active part in planning and carrying out activities with their parents. For the first meeting, the children's group might make a list of helpful things their parents do such as "My parents listen to me even when I stutter," or "My dad makes sure my brother doesn't interrupt me when I'm talking." This list then can be shared by the children when the groups meet together, and it will likely encourage discussion.

The parents group will also come up with activities for the combined meetings. One of our parent groups learned about how the right and left sides of the brain might be working in stuttering. They presented these ideas, accompanied by drawings, to the children when the two groups met together; and a lively discussion ensued.

Subsequent Meetings of the Children's Group. Experience has taught us how many activities to plan for the group in the time we have. In our hour-long meetings, we usually plan two or three activities and keep an eye on the clock so we can finish the most important activities before the parents join us. Some activities or

---

[1] We recommend Rebecca Zafir's book *The Zen of Listening* (2000) as a guide to help clinicians develop the ability to listen.

topics we may focus on only once. Others we may revisit again and again, for example:

- teasing
- bullying
- voluntary stuttering
- releasing feelings
- talking with parents
- talking with siblings and friends

In general, every session includes time for sharing and relationship building, fluency practice, and emotional release. Some of our activities will combine several of these components.

With a new group, one early focus is helping children learn what they do when they talk and what they do when they stutter. We use a painted plywood profile of a person's head and torso to depict the lips, tongue, jaw, voice-box, and lungs. We play games that help children learn the parts of their speech mechanism. We help them learn some of the things they do when they stutter, such as "squeezing at my voice-box" or "pushing hard with my tongue."

Through this activity, children learn some of the physical things they do when they stutter, talk about their stuttering, teach others to stutter like they do, feel what they are doing when they are right in the middle of a stutter. Then they are able to step back from the embarrassment, shame, and guilt that normally swallow them up when they stutter. Getting free of the shackles of these feelings will allow children the freedom to talk whether they stutter or not. Often some of the children immediately talk with far less stuttering. Others may take several weeks to show change. We work on this over several sessions and with lots of different games and activities. These activities are selected so that the children have fun while they work on their stuttering. This is crucial to make the hard work palatable. It is also a good idea to use games and activities that allow the children to show off their skills and knowledge. This helps them feel competent as they work on their stuttering because stuttering has made them feel helpless in the past.

Throughout the semester, we take the children through various activities to help them release their feelings. An early activity might be to have every child think of a time they really hated their stuttering or a time when a listener was difficult. Then they write down on toilet paper a word or two or a drawing depicting the experience and as a group, they flush the paper down a nearby toilet. Other activities we've used to release feelings include drawing pictures of stuttering, writing and acting out a play, and popping balloons with "stutters" painted on them.

Another powerful activity is voluntary stuttering. We always explain to the group why we are asking them to do voluntary or purposeful stuttering[2]. Our major rationale is that it makes us less afraid of stuttering and therefore we don't physically tense our muscles as much when we stutter. When we stutter in a more relaxed way, it feels better and sounds more like regular speech. Voluntary stuttering can really turn the tables on the avoidances that children have usually developed and it can give them a feeling of control over their stuttering. As we work on voluntary stuttering, we use plenty of games and activities that promote friendly competition among teams. We make up rules that reward voluntary stutters, such as requiring children to stutter when they take a turn or rewarding a high number of voluntary stutters by the teams with a pizza, skating, or bowling party at the end of the semester.

We begin teaching voluntary stuttering by showing the group some mild repetitions, and we use tokens or other tangible reinforcers to reward children who use purposeful stuttering in their speech. Once the group is good at voluntary stuttering, we encourage children to use it while making phone calls together. We make real phone calls for things we actually need or want to know about. Sometimes we order a pizza for the group; before placing the order, we might check prices at various pizza places. Sometimes we need to find out when stores at the mall close or when a bowling alley can schedule the whole group. We also make calls to ask for a particular CD or book, to find out the price of a dozen bagels, or to determine how much a tattoo of Britney Spears' name would cost. We always rehearse these calls before

---

[2] Carl Dell's book *Treating the School-Age Child Who Stutters* (Stuttering Foundation Publication No. 0014) has some good suggestions about voluntary stuttering in a section called "Making Stuttering More Voluntary."

making them, practicing just where we'll put in voluntary stuttering. Sometimes the group members make signs to display during the calls, like "Great going!" We use a speaker phone so everyone can hear both sides of the call. It is truly impressive to see a group of 5 or 6 children absolutely silent, holding up signs of encouragement and giving the thumbs-up to the speaker during these calls. Of course, much of the stuttering is real, because a telephone call to a stranger can be a difficult task for a child.

Little by little, with practice and encouragement, the stuttering with which children formerly felt helpless becomes something they can change. One of our sister groups in another city has introduced a contest to see which child can produce the longest purposeful stutter, the loudest one, the easiest one, the hardest, and the most spectacular. They have even had as a guest a circuit court judge who stutters, who arrives in full regalia to judge their stuttering contests.

After voluntary stuttering has been practiced and each child is accomplished at it, we teach the following fluency skills:

- slow rate
- easy onsets
- proprioception (feeling what you are doing)
- staying in the stutter until reducing tension so that the stutter is loose and voluntary at the end.[3]

We also teach pragmatic skills, such as natural eye contact, appropriate volume, listening and turn-taking that help make interactions successful. We practice these skills in small groups of one or two children. Sometimes they describe an experience or share how they feel with one other child, but not with the whole group. When the children seem to have learned skills in the small group, we encourage them use these skills in the whole group. This requires very structured activities with lots of support.

Sometimes children can use fluency skills in the parent-child group, especially when we have these children teaching the skills

---

[3] These fluency skills and others are described for children in our book *Easy Talker* (Pro-Ed).

to their parents. With group support, some of the children are able to use their skills during phone calls. After we have met for six or eight weeks and the children have learned to use voluntary stuttering and fluency skills, we take trips to the mall, the library or a candy store so that they can practice speaking. With permission from our listeners, we videotape some of the encounters and show the tapes when the groups meet together.

Subsequent Meetings of the Parents' Group. The content of the meetings of the parent group are much more determined by the parents than by us. We then let them decide if and when they would like to have a presentation or discussion on a particular topic. For example, most groups would like information on what the possible causes of stuttering are. One parent group made up visual aids to present the information about the causes. At the parents' request we bring in a variety of speakers, such as the head of the state speech-language-hearing association who discussed parents' rights and ways to obtain special education services for their child. At another time, a classroom teacher who stutters visited the parent group and talked about how parents can help their child and his teachers communicate about the problem. She also discussed how parents can work with teachers to respond to teasing and bullying.

In our parents' group, we always introduce the voluntary stuttering and fluency skills that the children are learning.[4] There are two reasons for this. First, this lets the parents know what the children are learning. Second, because the children will later be teaching these strategies to their parents, it gives the parents a chance to be comfortable with them. In our experience, parents sometimes feel uncomfortable when their children ask them to stutter on purpose. Occasionally the parent is also a person who stutters, but even these parents need to learn to voluntarily stutter in an easy, relaxed manner. When we train parents in voluntary stuttering, the experience of the children teaching their parents to stutter is less anxiety-producing and more satisfying. The meetings during which we teach parents to be at ease while voluntarily

---

[4] If a parent really does not want to stutter voluntarily, we do not push them to do it. So far none of the parents in our groups has refused to do so.

stuttering produce considerable discussion of feelings among the parents. This provides a valuable opportunity to explore how parents react to stuttering in general and their own child's in particular. Parents will probably have very different feelings than their children do about voluntary stuttering and this provides a topic for discussion in both the parent group and the combined group.

Subsequent Meetings of the Combined Group. In the combined group it is common for the children to prepare a topic to share with their parents. For example, when the children learn about how they produce speech, they share this information with their parents, using a plywood model of the speech mechanism. They then ask their parents to guess the parts of the mechanism used to produce various sounds. As a by-product of this activity, parents sometimes comment they are surprised to hear how much fluent speech their children exhibit, compared to the relatively small amount of stuttering.

In another example, the children used the meeting of the combined group to teach their parents to stutter. Sometimes the activity is for children to teach their parent how to stutter like they do. At these times the children grade their parents on their various attempts to stutter. We facilitate as needed, ensuring that each parent-child pair has a good experience and that the group is supportive of every attempt.

At some point, when the children and parents seem ready, the combined group can have contests and judge who, among both parents and children, can produce the longest, funniest, or easiest stutters. In addition, the children guide their parents in phone calls using voluntary stutters and fluency skills. Toward the end of the year or semester, the combined group will go to a shopping mall and use voluntary stutters and fluency skills. One of us takes the parents and the other takes the children on expeditions to different shops in the mall. Afterwards, parent-child pairs go out to voluntarily stutter and use fluency skills. Later, we all meet at a restaurant to compare experiences. These adventures help the parents understand what sorts of listener reactions their child has to cope with, thus increasing the parent's respect and empathy for the child, bringing them closer together.

An important result of group therapy—especially when the groups are combined—is that the parents hear their children talk about things that might never be discussed at home. Many of the children's groups have helped their parents understand what is helpful and what is not. For example, some children have requested feedback or reminders from parents about their stuttering, whereas other children have said that that is the last thing they want. Many parents have reported that the meeting has stimulated great conversations about stuttering in the car on the way home.

Group Therapy in a School Setting

Some of our colleagues have used group therapy for children in school settings. For example, a clinician who works with high school students brings together four teens from different schools every other week. The guidance counselor from one of the schools helps her run the group. The structure and activities for this older group are different from those in our younger groups, but the goals are much the same. Often discussion is started by a student sharing an experience he's had during the past week. Other times a video about stuttering or a guest participant will kick off lively conversation. As the teens share their feelings about their stuttering and experiences they've had, they feel less alone and are able to accept these feelings. As a result, these emotions become less intense and self-acceptance develops, making stuttering easier to change. Every session includes some direct work on stuttering as well as some exploration and sharing of feelings. Occasionally, but not often, the clinician brings the teens' parents into a combined group to promote communication about stuttering.

Group work with younger children in a school setting is similar to the group therapy we've described in this chapter. A major difference is that it is difficult for most parents of these children to meet on a regular basis during the school day. It may be possible to have parents come to an occasional parent group meeting. This can take place in the evening when parent-teacher association meetings take place or parent-teacher conferences are held. It may also be possible to meet in the late afternoon if the school system is willing to let the clinician work on a flexible schedule. If parent meetings are infrequent, it is important to use the time available to have parents share their feelings with each other so they can feel mutual support.

We have presented only a few examples of how groups can be structured. Other clinicians may lead groups in entirely different ways, with greater emphasis on expressing feelings or more time spent practicing fluency and communication skills. Regardless, we feel that a major outcome of group therapy should always be that children feel increased kinship with others who stutter and are better able to manage their stuttering on their own.

Bibliography

Bloodstein, O. (1995). *A handbook on stuttering.* San Diego: Singular Publishing Group, Inc.

Conture, E. (2001). *Stuttering: Its nature, diagnosis, and treatment.* Boston: Allyn and Bacon.

Dell, C. (2010). *Treating the School-Age Child Who Stutters: A guide for clinicians.* Second edition. (Stuttering Foundation Publication No. 0014). Memphis: Stuttering Foundation of America.

Guitar, B. (1998). *Stuttering: An integrated approach to its nature and treament.* Baltimore: Lippincott, Williams, & Wilkins.

Guitar, B. and Reville, J. (1997). *Easy talker: A fluency workbook for school-age children.* Austin, TX: Pro-Ed.

Lewis,M. and Haviland-Jones, J. (2000). *Handbook of emotions.* NY: Guilford Press.

Luterman, D. (2001). *Counseling persons with communication disorders and their families.* Austin, TX: Pro-Ed.

Shafir, R. (2000). *The Zen of listening.* Wheaton, IL: Quest Books.

Van Riper, C. (1982). *The nature of stuttering.* Englewood Cliffs, N.J.: Prentice Hall.

Further Reading

Conture, E. and Melnick, K. (1999). Parent-child group approach to stuttering in preschool and school-age children. In M. Onslow and A. Packman (Eds.) *Early stuttering: A handbook of intervention strategies.* (pp. 17-51) San Diego, CA: Singular Publishing.

Gregory, H. (2003). *Stuttering therapy: Rationale and procedures.* Boston: Allyn and Bacon.

Kelly, E. and Conture, E. (1991). Intervention with school-age stutterers: A parent-child fluency group approach. *Seminars in speech and language,* 12 (4) 309-321.

Logan, K. & Caruso, A. (1997). Parents as partners in the treatment of childhood stuttering. *Seminars in speech and language,* 18 (4) 309 - 327.

Logan, K. & Yaruss, S. (1999). Helping parents address attitudinal and emotional factors with young children who stutter. *Contemporary issues in communication science and disorders,* 26, 69-81.

Zebrowski, P. & Kelly, E. (2002). *Manual of stuttering intervention.* Clifton Park, NY: Singular Publishing Group.

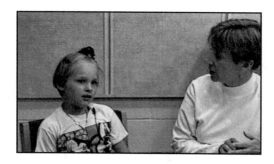

Chapter **8**

understanding and coping with emotions: counseling teenagers who stutter

Patricia M. Zebrowski, Ph.D.

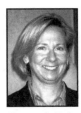 For most adults in any kind of helping profession (e.g. teachers, psychologists, speech-language pathologists, etc.) working with teenagers offers a unique set of challenges. The "adolescent mandate" (Wolfe, 1991) to simultaneously let go of childhood, yet retain the feelings of safety and comfort that (hopefully) define this period of life, creates fairly consistent turmoil for both the teen and his or her family—ranging from very intense to low-grade. When adults in the adolescent's life attempt to teach, guide, instruct, advise—all those things we do as parents, teachers or counselors—we almost always find the going rough. The intellectual, emotional and physical changes and confusion that characterize the teenage years frequently make teens resistant or uninterested in what we have to teach them. As a result, it is often the case that teens are dismissed from therapy or counseling because they are deemed "unmotivated" to continue. While that certainly appears true in many cases, at least on the surface, I propose that being "unmotivated" is actually a place to start, not

end. What are the behaviors or comments that we see that make us regard the teen as unmotivated? Are there alternative explanations for what we perceive as lack of motivation? Unmotivated to do what? What's so bad about being unmotivated?

This space between the proverbial "rock and a hard place" is where we often find ourselves when we want to help teenagers. For adolescents who stutter, this uncomfortable space is shared with the behavior of stuttering and all its associated emotions, thoughts, and attitudes. In this chapter, I will describe ways in which speech-language pathologists can stay in that space with the teenager who stutters and help him or her to recognize the choices that lie beyond it.

Counseling Methods

Luterman (2001) states that when speech-language pathologists and audiologists "counsel" their clients, they most frequently do so by informing and persuading. In the first, the client is provided with information about the problem, the diagnosis, and recommendations for intervention, if necessary. In the second, the clinician conveys to the client that as the expert, he or she knows what is best for the client in the way of treatment options. As Luterman notes, the underlying assumption of this approach is that the clinician possesses all of the relevant information and knowledge, and the client possesses none (or, at least, an inadequate amount). Therefore, the clinician is capable of making better decisions for the clients than the clients can make for themselves.

As clinicians working with teenagers who stutter, our attempts to teach, guide, instruct and advise boil down to informing and persuading (Luterman, 2001; Gregory, 1983). And as previously discussed, such methods frequently lead to resistance or apathy in the adolescent, and thus, our decision that they are unmotivated, and not 'ready' for therapy. In actuality, this is most likely true...they are not ready for or open to this type of therapy. Luterman states that:

"These two counseling approaches—counseling by informing and counseling by persuading—are not mutually exclusive. There are components of both in most (inadequate) counseling sessions. After first informing the client of test results (and treatment options), we often set about convincing him or her of what to do about the data. A combination of informing and persuading counseling strategies can be very potent. When we *overwhelm* (italics mine) with information, we also undermine the client's confidence...(p. 5)."

Considered within the context of the "adolescent mandate" described earlier, it's no wonder that teenagers are often unresponsive to our attempts to help them. We run the risk that they perceive our attempts to inform and persuade (i.e. teach) them as evidence that they are not being heard.

A third approach to counseling discussed by Luterman is that of *listening and valuing*. According to Luterman, in this approach, the client (here, the teenager who stutters) is viewed as competent to make good decisions, and our role as speech-language pathologists is to use our specialized knowledge to point the client toward the paths that are possible.

Listening and Valuing:
Feelings Associated With Stuttering

Considering that stuttering is usually a disorder that begins in early childhood, it is safe to assume that most adolescents who stutter have been doing so for many years. As such, they exhibit 'persistent stuttering' (Yairi and Ambrose, 1999) of a more chronic, less variable form. Their experiences with stuttering over time typically lead to a wide variety of emotions, and related learned, reactive behavior, as discussed by Gregory (Chapter 1) and Guitar (Chapter 5). Thus, when we work with teens, we need to recognize that the speech behaviors of stuttering, that is, the repetitions, blocks and prolongations of sounds, represent one 'level' of the problem - a level that can be influenced by thoughts and emotions. In order to begin to peel away the cognitive and affective layers of stuttering, the adolescent needs to have a safe environment in which he or she can identify and label thoughts and feelings, and see how they are related not only to each other, but to the behavior they might trigger. This behavior might be speech specific, for example, initiating a sound or word with excessive laryngeal tension when stuttering is anticipated, or using repetitive interjections (i.e. "uh" or "well") prior to the production of a word that is 'felt' to be hard to say fluently. Or, it can be relatively general, such as avoiding speech situations or ordering something in a restaurant because it is "easy to say", rather than because it is what one wants. The important point is that when teenagers can recognize a feeling and objectively view the behavior that stems from it, they can start to explore ways to change this seemingly automatic relationship. How does this happen?

One way is through the use of cognitive restructuring, a method that employs both *listening and valuing,* but also *questioning.* Cognitive restructuring is based on the "cognitive model," which considers a person's perception of self, of others, and of the world, as the primary influence on emotions, and subsequently, behavior (Beck, 1995; Zebrowski, 2002).

According to Beck, there is a hierarchical relationship between beliefs and behavior, in which a person's core beliefs (i.e. those that develop in early childhood and are deeply ingrained and often unarticulated) give rise to intermediate beliefs, which finally yield automatic thoughts, emotions and behaviors. Many teenagers are

...there is a hierarchical relationship between beliefs and behavior...

unable to recognize, let alone label, the feelings they are experiencing. For some of these adolescents, one way to help them develop an awareness of their emotions is to start by asking them to identify automatic thoughts, and tie them to the feelings with which they may coincide.

Automatic thoughts reflect a "stream of thinking" that occurs simultaneously with more readily or apparent or perceived thoughts (Beck, 1964; Beck, 1995). For the most part, we are relatively unaware of our automatic thoughts; they tend to be fleeting, perhaps surfacing into our consciousness for a few seconds and then submerging again. What we are aware of, however, is the feeling or emotion that they may trigger, although we are typically unable to identify the feeling. Rather, we are aware of autonomic nervous system arousal and the resulting physiological feelings that follow (e.g. dry mouth, increased heart rate, "butterflies" in the stomach, and so forth).

As an example, when I am teaching a class, I may be aware of thoughts related to the material I'm trying to convey and how to clearly convey it. Simultaneously, I may entertain a fleeting, automatic thought that the "students don't like me." This may trigger an emotional response—at least I'm aware that my face is getting red, and my palms are sweating—and at the time, or later, I may appreciate this feeling as "embarrassment" or "shame" or some other emotion. These emotions, if chronic, may lead me to start avoiding teaching or interacting with students. On the other hand, if I can be objective, I can question the validity and usefulness of the thoughts that stem from these emotions.

How do I start using this strategy with teens who stutter? First and foremost, I listen to their stories and value what they tell me, and I make the effort to establish a trusting relationship based on mutual respect. Eventually, I increase the number of **open** ("Why are you here today?") or **closed** ("Is talking hard or easy for you? Is it hard sometimes, and easy at other times?") questions I ask. During our conversations, I look for what Beck (1995) described as an "affect shift", such as a change in facial expression, eye-gaze or posture, or a verbal cue such as a pitch, tone or volume change while talking. When these shifts are observed, I ask "What was going through your mind just then?" If the teen says "nothing" (a common response, at first), I nod and move on. Here it is a good idea to use an "advance-retreat-advance" approach (Zebrowski, 2002), in that I move on when the teen is noncommittal, and use his or her subsequent comments to form a bridge back to the original question. For example, if a teen tells me that his stuttering doesn't bother him, I might recall for him an earlier comment in which he stated that he avoided school dances because he knew he would have to talk.

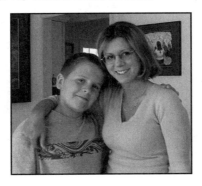

As I continue to try to elicit these "hot cognitions" (Beck, 1995), at some point the teen will be able to recognize an automatic thought that is likely to be related in some way to speaking or stuttering. Examples might include: "I was thinking that I can't say it", or "I'm going to stutter," "You think I'm not smart," and so on. Once these and similar thoughts have been identified, the adolescent can tie an emotion to the thought. For example, if the teen becomes aware of thinking "I can't do it" when speaking in class, perhaps the associated emotion is fear, or fear of embarrassment. And, after examining these automatic thought-emotion relationships, the teenager may come to realize that the "I can't do it" thought can trigger something as general as reticence to speak, or something as specific as cessation of airflow and increased laryngeal tension (Zebrowski, 2002).

Using this approach to help teenagers recognize and label their feelings can open a door to talk about these emotions. By listening in an open, nonjudgmental way, I can provide teens with a supportive context in which they can problem-solve ways to separate *feelings* from unproductive *behaviors*.

Emotions of Stuttering

Obviously, each teen will experience unique feelings, but there are some emotions that are more frequently experienced by adolescents who stutter as a group. These include feeling isolated or alone, confused, helpless, guilty, anxious, ashamed, embarrassed, or afraid. While it is most important to listen, affirm and help teens recognize the connection between what they *feel* and *do* (i.e. the link between emotions and behavior), we can also do the following things to defuse strong negative emotions.

Feelings of isolation. Since the prevalence of stuttering is relatively low, it is not unusual for teens who stutter to never see, meet or talk with another person (let alone another adolescent) who stutters. This situation often contributes to strong feelings of isolation which can affect a number of areas such as socialization and social-emotional development. An important thing we can do for teens—and others, for that matter—who stutter is to introduce them to other teenagers who stutter, either formally in a support or therapy group, or informally through a social venue. In this publication, Drs. Ramig and Guitar offer suggestions for group work with both adults and children who stutter. These same principles are also appropriate for teens. In addition, when I establish a strong relationship with a teenager, I convey to the teen that he or she is not "alone in the boat" (Zebrowski and Schum, 1993). One very important point here is that it is the *relationship,* and the *quality and the consistency of the relationship* between the clinician and the teen that is key in helping the teen to manage feelings of isolation and their resultant behavior. The speech modification strategies that are taught in therapy, or the success or lack of success the teen has in using them, really has little to do with changing the feeling the adolescent may have of being alone. In her book, *Chasing Grace* (1996), psychologist Martha Manning describes the importance of this relationship:

> "It has taken me years past my clinical training as a psychologist to realize that no matter how good I am, I can't lessen the number of miles on the road, even for people I love like crazy. I can't walk that long way for them. But, I know that just having a companion on some part of the road can make the long, lonely walk seem shorter, and make the journey, however difficult, infinitely more bearable (p. 100.)"

Feelings of confusion and helplessness. Typically, teenagers struggle with feelings of confusion about what stuttering is, why they stutter, and what they can do about it. These confused feelings often lead to feelings of helplessness, or of being overwhelmed. "Learned helplessness", which Seligman (1998) describes as the "giving-up reaction, or the quitting response that follows from the belief that whatever you do doesn't matter (p. 15)" also frequently comes into play here. It's my speculation that what is perceived as the teen's lack of motivation masks the face of their confusion, learned helplessness, and their feelings of being overwhelmed. In addition to helping teenagers identify emotions and tie them to behavior, I also provide them with:

- current information about what stuttering is and is not, expressed in an easy-to-understand fashion;
- a clear explanation of the different approaches to stuttering treatment that are available to them;
- speech modification strategies early on in therapy, making sure to highlight to the teen the ways in which he or she has been able to make speech change (no matter how small).

In this regard, I make sure to choose strategies that have the highest probability of being relatively quickly learned and successfully used by the teen.

Guilt and shame. Guilt and shame are two related but different emotions that can typically accompany persistent stuttering. As experts have previously distinguished them, (Sheehan, 1982, in Chapter 3; Murphy, 1998), *guilt* is the discomfort or pain that comes from doing something we regret, while *shame* is the discomfort or pain that comes from believing that a part of us is defective, or bad. Guilt comes from what we *do;* shame comes from what we *are.* As such, while the things we *do* that cause us to feel guilty can be "fixed" (thus eliminating guilt), the things we *are* that cause us to feel shame cannot.

For teenagers who stutter, guilt can be the result of misinformation or lack of information about stuttering, particularly with regard to what caused stuttering to begin when they were younger. If adolescents believe that there is something that they *did* that caused stuttering, then it is likely that guilty feelings about these (perhaps unknown but guessed-at) actions will arise. In addition, due to the variability that is inherent to childhood stuttering, friends and family members often convey to the teenager that he or she could stop stuttering (or at least "control it") if they wanted. To help teens manage these feelings of guilt, I find it useful to consider guilt as a form of anxiety (Zebrowski and Schum, 1993). In this way, I use the strategies of *reassurance, focusing* and *binding,* which together can assist in coping with guilty feelings. In *reassurance,* I let the teen know that (1) they are not "alone in the boat" and (2) that stuttering is such a complex problem that no single action or event is sufficient to 'cause' stuttering. Through *focusing,* I help teens find a specific concern that can be addressed, such as using 'smooth' speech during introductions, or dealing with parents. This focus on a single issue helps them attend to the here and now, rather than persist in shifting between the past (What did I do to cause stuttering?), and the future (What will happen if I always stutter?). It is this continual shifting between past and future worries that fuels anxiety and guilt. Finally, in using *binding activities,* I give the teenager something to do that will serve to tie up any free-floating anxiety and help to retain focus on the here and now. Giving homework and reading assignments is obviously an excellent way to do this.

Managing feelings of shame is much less straightforward. How does one eliminate a negative feeling when it is related to something one is, something that is part of one's constitution, and thus, cannot be changed? Feelings of shame often lead to maladaptive or nonproductive behaviors, and through listening, affirming and cognitive restructuring, I can help the teen recognize those relationships. I can also hope to directly influence the adolescent's belief system by helping him to:

- recognize that stuttering is something one does, not something one has because of something one is (Williams, 1957; 1979);
- become desensitized to stuttering through talking about it, exploring general issues of speaking, and accepting that it is normal to make mistakes; and
- use purposeful or voluntary stuttering as a way to see that stuttering is a behavior that can be managed

Embarrassment. Feeling embarrassed is a part of adolescence. It stems from a number of sources, but often is most strongly related to being "different" and standing out from what is considered 'normal' or 'cool' or both! Certainly teenagers who stutter are different from other teens in the way they speak, and that, of course can be an added source of embarrassment, added to the embarrassed feelings that arise from not having the right clothes, having a 'bad hair' day, acne, parents, siblings, and so on. Cognitive restructuring, as described earlier, is an excellent way of managing embarrassment, as well as the fear of being embarrassed. Once the adolescent has identified the feeling of embarrassment, I help them evaluate both the *validity* and *usefulness* of the *automatic thoughts* that yield embarrassed feelings. As Beck (1995) describes, one of the best ways to do this is through a series of questions that might include:

What evidence do I have to support this idea?

What is the worst thing that could happen *if this were true?*

What is the best thing that could happen?

What is the effect of my believing this thought?

What could be the effect of *changing* my thinking?

What should I do about it?

What would I tell a friend if he or she had the same thought?

It can be very helpful for teens to keep a journal or diary to record the automatic thoughts that trigger embarrassment (typically surrounding specific events or situations), and then to have them record the observed outcome as a way to assess the validity of these thoughts.

Fear. For many teens who stutter, fear starts out being specific to speaking and stuttering but can then become more generalized to encompass things like social interaction and almost anything that involves risk-taking. Unfortunately, it is the willingness to take risks, small or large, that is important to the reduction or elimination of fear. The speech-language pathologist who works with teenagers who stutter needs to recognize the importance of promoting risk-taking as a way to manage feelings of fear. Starting out by encouraging small, but salient risk (i.e. the teens ability to disclose an emotion during therapy) and pointing out to the teen the victory in doing it is an excellent way to start. Adolescents who are willing and able to use purposeful or voluntary stuttering are taking a healthy risk, and for many, this venture is a major step in eliminating fear. Generalization of risk-taking behavior to such things as self-disclosure (letting listeners know you are a person who stutters), engaging in speaking situations at higher and higher levels of difficulty, and *just talking more* are also powerful things to do to decrease fear. Our role as clinicians is to help teens who stutter approach increasingly difficult tasks with confidence, providing lots of coaching and encouragement along the way.

Bibliography

Beck, J.S. (1995). *Cognitive therapy. Basics and beyond.* New York: The Guilford Press.

Luterman, D.M. (2001). *Counseling Persons with Communication Disorders and Their Families* (4th ed). Austin, TX: Pro-ed.

Manning, M. (1996). *Chasing Grace. Reflections of a Catholic Girl, Grown Up.* San Francisco: Harper.

Seligman, M.E.P. (1998) *Learned Optimism. How to Change Your Mind and Your Life.* New York: Pocket Books.

Wolf, A.E. (1991). *"Get out of my life, but first could you drive me and Cheryl to the mall?" A parent's guide to the new teenager.* New York: The Noonday Press.

Yairi, E., and Ambrose, N.G. (1999). Early Childhood Stuttering I: Persistency and Recovery Rates. *Journal of Speech, Language, and Hearing Research,* 42(5), 1097-1112.

Zebrowski, P.M., and Schum, R.L. (1993). Counseling parents of children who stutter. *American Journal of Speech-Language Pathology,* 2(2), 65-73.

Chapter **9**

counseling adults in group therapy

Peter R. Ramig, Ph.D.

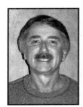 In chapter 3 of this book, Dr. Joseph Sheehan masterfully describes how shame and guilt can fuel the use of avoidances that lead to the continuation, and even worsening, of the problem of adult stuttering. He concludes his chapter with a listing of counseling principles pertinent to successful intervention with persons who stutter.

In this chapter, I will draw from my experience at the University of Colorado, and that of my graduate clinicians, in conducting group intervention over several years with adults who stutter. In my experience, many of these individuals fit the profile, defined by Cooper, (1997) as "chronic perseverative stuttering." This classification includes those persons whose "stuttering syndrome consists of multiple and coexisting and interactive affective, behavioral, and cognitive components coalescing over a period of years." This population includes those needing to deal with the issues of fear, shame, guilt and frustration as described by Dr. Sheehan in his chapter. These feelings develop as a consequence of years of trying to suppress and avoid stuttering. Although a complete cure is remote with this population, many are capable of improving significantly by learning they can stutter with less effort, fewer avoidances, and more confidence in their approach to speaking. My focus in this chapter includes a cadre of principles pertaining to group intervention, and the inseparable role counseling plays in that process. My views on group counseling are in line with Cooper's definition of counseling as a process through which individuals participate in the "mutual exploration" of beliefs, attitudes, and feelings (Cooper, 1992). For additional information on group support and counseling of adults who stutter, the reader is directed to Ramig and Bennett (1997).

The Importance of Group Therapy

Why is group therapy an essential component in the management of stuttering? Experience over the years confirms our belief that group intervention with adults who stutter is more a necessity than an option (Ramig and Bennett, 1997). Most advantageous is the intensive structured speech practice that takes place with the cooperative involvement of several clients in a more real-life environment. Because of this, the group provides excellent practice opportunities when compared to non-group intervention programs.

The group experience facilitates the development of a sense of belonging in an atmosphere of unconditional positive regard (Rollin, 1987). Group structure allows for a variety of viewpoints and experiences, facilitating a better understanding of the complexities of stuttering and the negative life impact (e.g. Van Riper, 1973) often associated with the experience of chronic stuttering. These benefits can lead to better management of stuttering in real-life situations and can reduce the feelings of isolation and helplessness (Ramig and Bennett, 1997)

The Structure of Group Therapy with Adults

What is the structure and what are the required skills necessary to participate in our group therapy? Our groups typically consist of young adults in their early twenties to older clients ranging in age to the mid sixties. Most have stuttered since early childhood, are moderate to severe, and exhibit chronic stuttering. In addition, most have a prior therapy history, either working individually with a clinician, and/or in one or more of the intensive stuttering programs. Our sessions are held once a week for 90 minutes, with a maximum of six clients assigned to each group.

With rare exception, all participants must first complete one or more semesters of individual stuttering treatment in our University of Colorado Speech and Hearing Center. This first step is necessary because of our expectations of skill level and performance for each and every client. For example, to be successful in group intervention, clients must first learn the rudiments of using specific fluency enhancing and modification of stuttering strategies in individual treatment. Every participant, including clinicians, must be able to accurately implement the fluency shaping procedures of easy onsets, light contacts, relaxation, and

...stuttering is a daily reality negatively impacting life...

rate control, as well as more confrontational stuttering modification techniques of **pre-block, in-block** and **post-block corrections,** and voluntary stuttering. Also included in their training are intensive motor practice and behavioral awareness of what they do when they stutter and how they interfere with normal speech production. For many of our clients, past attempts to manage stuttering solely by trying "not to stutter" have been unsuccessful. For this reason, we believe it is necessary to provide tools to confront and work through stuttering without the effortful pushing, forcing and struggling. It is our belief that it is best to provide the client with strategies to both reduce stuttering through fluency shaping strategies and stuttering modification techniques. As described by Guitar (1998), combining and emphasizing both "schools" of thought can be an effective way to better enable those who stutter.

For many clients, stuttering is a daily reality that negatively impacts their life. Therefore, it is necessary to teach strategies to encourage a way of stuttering that is less effortful and more forward flowing. With these tools in hand, they then join the group and embark on speaking activities that reflect everyday communication experiences. In that regard, the main purpose of our adult group is to facilitate transfer and maintenance activities in an environment of support, encouragement and acceptance, while maintaining expectations that encourage change.

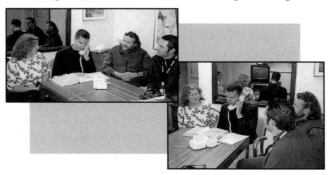

Group Management Skills

What skills are necessary to effectively manage a group? One of the most important responsibilities in managing group intervention is to present content that is meaningful (e.g. Jacobs, Harvill and Masson, 1988; Ramig and Bennett, 1997; and Shames, 2000). This includes choosing activities that are appropriate, important, and attainable to individuals and group members collectively. To accomplish this goal, we must be skillful and assertive in:

- taking charge and directing individuals and the group;
- actively listening and attending;
- being silent when appropriate;
- reflecting and clarifying;
- "cutting-off" members who abuse talking time;
- making sure every member participates equally;
- "drawing-out" those who may be less talkative or prone to participate;
- freely modeling fluency shaping and stuttering modification techniques expected of clients.

Taking charge and directing individuals and the group.
Directing a group of adults can initially be intimidating for even the more experienced clinician. This is especially the case for graduate clinicians lacking experience in conducting group intervention with those who stutter. In that regard, all of our 'new' groups which start at the beginning of a semester include a graduate clinician who, in the previous semester, co-directed one of the adult groups. In the following semester, that same person, now experienced, is paired with and serves as a mentor to a clinician lacking experience, and who then becomes gradually more involved in the planning and implementation of sessions. However, with a well-planned, organized agenda, initial feelings of discomfort typically transform into positive anticipation of conducting subsequent sessions.

Active listening and attending. This is the counselor's vehicle to facilitating client comfort, one of the first ingredients leading to change. It is viewed as an important counseling component and skill (Burnard, 1992; Luterman, 1991; Ramig and Bennett, 1997; Rollin, 1987 and Shames, 2000). Included in this component is the clinician's demonstration of paying careful attention to content, voice, and body language. Listening intently to the content of the message includes attention to the client's exact words, use of phrases, and colloquialisms. In addition, vocal components of speech—including pitch, volume, and word stress—are possible indicators of the client's emotional status. Another component, body language or nonverbal communication, can be a very important clue to how the client is feeling at the moment. Included here are the client's facial expressions, gestures while speaking, and body posture and stance. Further, as Zebrowski describes in Chapter 8, changes in these can also indicate changes in the client's mood or thought. In turn, the cues given by the clinician to demonstrate active listening and attending include an open body position and stance, such as leaning forward, appropriate eye contact, and a relaxed demeanor (Burnard, 1992). Active listening is demonstrated by the clinician's use of head nodding, brief one-word confirmations such as "yes," "good," and "hmm."

Demonstrate appropriate silence. Using silence productively is another attribute of an effective clinician when demonstrating active listening. In fact, Luterman (2001) states that clinician silence in group intervention is probably the most important way to stimulate change. Specifically, Luterman notes that silence can serve to add some discomfort causing clients to speak up, thus facilitating a more active client role in group activities. In addition, he feels that appropriately timed silence aids in effectively cueing the group to move on to another topic and can also signal that it is time to terminate the group session. Doyle (1992) states that silence is an effective strategy to use whenever clients have difficulty expressing their thoughts as a result of feeling emotional, confused or stressed. These moments of silence serve as an indicator that we are interested, attentive and respectful of the clients' need to express himself.

Reflecting and clarifying. Although these are separate components, they often act in cooperative combination. Reflection involves our restatement of what we think the client has said. This can involve rewording the client's message to better ensure that the clinician and group members understand what was said. It can also include the clinician's adding a statement acknowledging client feelings and emotions. We can use clarification as a request to the client to restate a comment that may be unclear to one or more group participants. For example, if the client says "This is too hard!" we may say "What exactly is difficult for you? Do you mean it is hard to talk about stuttering?"

Cut-off clients who abuse talking time. Sometimes members of the group deviate from the topic at hand, talk incessantly, attempt to rescue[3] another member, and make inappropriate or attacking comments. At these times we need to stop and redirect the conversation. This may be accomplished indirectly by making eye contact with the client speaking and then diverting one's eyes to another in the group; or it may need to be more direct such as "Sarah, you may not agree with Justin, but let him express his thoughts." Although cutting-off strategies can be more confrontive, they are sometimes necessary for smooth and cohesive group function.[4]

---

[3] Rescuing is defined by Jacobs et al. (1988) as an attempt to "smooth over the negative emotions someone else is experiencing."

[4] In my experience, cutting-off strategies are the most difficult for beginning graduate students to apply, especially when clients are older than the clinician.

Cutting-off is also important in apportioning talking time in order to ensure there is time to address the activities planned for the session.

Drawing-out clients. This can be accomplished using both indirect or direct strategies. Simply initiating eye contact with the client you wish to engage is often enough to serve as a stimulus for him to respond. If necessary, once trust and positive rapport are established, we can use the more direct strategy of verbally inviting a reticent client to respond and become more active in the group.

Modeling skills. Fluency shaping and stuttering modification changes we expect our clients to implement to improve their stuttering can initially be difficult to learn and incorporate into everyday speech. For some clients resorting to the over-learned, undesirable behaviors is easier than using the newly-learned and more desirable patterns. Because even positive change can be difficult to establish and maintain, we require our clients and clinicians to model target behaviors throughout the group session. In order for our credibility to be strengthened, we should use in our own speech the same fluency enhancing and stuttering modification strategies expected of the clients. In contrast, our credibility can be seriously compromised if we are viewed as expecting from our clients that which we are unwilling or unable to model.

Disclosing The Obvious

For many, stuttering is a problem no one talks about. It becomes the dark shadow of the "unmentionable" that can fuel the feelings of shame and guilt in the speaker and create feelings of uneasiness in the listener because he is unsure how to respond. The listener ponders, should he say the word for the client, should he wait for him to get the word out, should he look away or maintain eye contact during the speaker's stuttering? These are some of the questions most listeners struggle with. Not only is the client embarrassed by his stuttering, but so is his listener. This can create a communication experience that is frustrating and uneasy for both. Talking, that communication process that is typically meant to be a positive interactive experience, becomes one of dread for the client and sometimes for the listener.

We believe the most debilitating aspect of the chronic syndrome stems from this need to avoid unavoidable stuttering (e.g. Agnello, 2003; Manning, 2003; Ramig, 2003; Sheehan, 1975 and 2003; Van Riper, 1973). The client tries diligently and often unsuccessfully not to stutter. Because adults who stutter often perceive that listeners view them as stupid, nervous, or emotionally unstable, they attempt to minimize the abnormality they feel by diligently and often unsuccessfully trying not to stutter.[5]

One of our goals in group intervention is for clients to discuss self-disclosure as a tool (eg. Molt, 2003; Manning, 2003; Molt, 2003; Murphy, 2003 and Ramig, 2003). We define self-disclosure as revealing to listeners that we stutter and that we may be practicing speech skills as we talk with them. Disclosing the obvious helps both the client and his listener feel more comfortable during communication. Disclosing addresses in a positive manner the fact stuttering is occurring and thus creates an opportunity for both speaker and listener to openly talk about it as the interesting (albeit frustrating) phenomenon it really is. Positive communication results through the listener now feeling more comfortable asking questions such as, "What causes stuttering?" "Why don't people stutter when they sing?" The listener also has the freedom to ask about the more acceptable ways to respond to a person who stutters when they are having difficulty.

Upon disclosing, the interaction typically transforms from one of distress, frustration, and embarrassment, to one that is more open and comfortable. It has been this writer's experience that most listeners are genuinely interested to learn more about the nature and treatment of stuttering. When the client discloses, he affords them the opportunity to ask questions and positively express their interest. This experience aids in mitigating the "dark side" of the "unmentionable," thereby paving the way for less stressful and positive communication for both. Finally, disclosing is an important ingredient in accomplishing the goal virtually all

---

[5]This is an overly simplistic explanation for a complex process. For more information on the avoidance of stuttering and suggestions for minimizing this need, the reader is encouraged to see The Stuttering Foundation publication, *Advice to Those Who Stutter* (second edition, 2011).

clients share: saying what they want to say when they want to say it, and doing so with less stuttering.

In our group, we introduce self-disclosure through activities designed to verbally address the fact that the person may be having a hard time talking. Specific wording is rehearsed in the group sessions by each member in several varied speaking situations, first within, and then outside of the treatment room. Through extensive practice, they are encouraged to develop wording that feels most comfortable to them. For example, during an awkward or embarrassing stuttering moment a client might decide to nonchalantly interject any one or combination of the following:

- "As you can see, I'm having a harder time controlling my stuttering today."

- "I'm needing to work on letting my stuttering come out more easily, bear with me while I work on doing so."

- "As a person who stutters, this is a more difficult speaking situation. Bear with me while I practice holding on to the sounds as I work through my dysfluencies."

- "I appreciate your wanting to help me say the words I'm getting stuck on, but I need the practice at saying them myself in a more easy manner than I have thus far."

- "I know my stuttering makes both of us uneasy sometimes, and that's certainly understandable, but I need to stretch out the sounds as I try to stutter in a forward flowing fashion. If I try to continue to hold it back or hide it in other ways, it just makes things worse. Thanks for being patient as I do my best to let it come out more easily."

- You've known me long enough to know that I stutter, and I've appreciated your sensitivity, attention, and patience. But if you have any questions about stuttering, feel free to ask. I'm glad to answer them as best I know."

The fact the client is able to disclose what he views as his nemesis lessens his need to hide and avoid stuttering, thus dissipating some of his stress and subsequent muscle tension that can otherwise exacerbate the problem. In addition, openly addressing stuttering affords the client an opportunity to state his need to work on his new fluency-enhancing and stuttering modification techniques he may otherwise have felt reluctant to practice. Disclosure now gives both the client and the listener "permission" to openly talk about stuttering and creates a more comfortable environment for the client to practice his strategies in his group intervention.

Bibliography

Alm, P. (1995). Study groups for stutterers—A valuable part of stuttering therapy? In C. W. Starkweather and H.F.M. Peters (eds.), *Stuttering: Proceedings of the first world congress on fluency disorders.* Nijmegen, the Netherlands: University Press Nijmegen.

Burnard, P. (1992). *Counseling skills training: A sourcebook of activities for trainers.* London, GB: Kogan Page Limited.

Cooper, E. B. (1997). Fluency disorders. In Thomas A. Crowe (Ed.), *Applications of counseling in speech-language pathology and audiology,* (pp 145–166). Baltimore, MD: Williams & Wilkins.

Conture, E.G. (2001). *Stuttering: Its nature, diagnosis, and treatment.* Boston, MA: Allyn and Bacon.

Doyle, R.E. (1992). *Essential skills and strategies in the helping process.* Pacific Grove, CA: Brooks/Cole Publishing Co.

Guitar, B. (1998). *Stuttering: An integrated approach to its nature and treatment* (2nd ed.). Baltimore, MD: Williams and Wilkins.

Jacobs, E.E., Harvill, R.L., and Masson, R.L. (1988). *Group counseling: Strategies and skills.* Belmont, CA: Wadsworth, Inc.

Luterman, D.M. (1991). *Counseling the communicatively disordered and their families.* Austin, TX: Pro-Ed.

Ramig, P.R. and Bennett, E.M. (1997). Considerations for conducting group intervention with adults who stutter. *Seminars in speech and language,* 18,(4), 343–356.

Rollin, W.J. (1987). *The psychology of communication disorders in individuals and their families.* Englewood Cliffs, NJ: Prentice-Hall.

Shames, G.S. (2000). *Counseling the communicatively disabled and their families: A manual for clinicians.* Boston, MA: Allyn & Bacon.

Simon, A.M. (1995). Therapeutic groups for adult stutterers. In C.W. Starkweather & H.F.M. Peters (eds.), *Stuttering: Proceedings of the first world congress on fluency disorders.* Nijmegen, the Netherlands: University Press Nijmegen.

Van Riper, C. (1973). *The treatment of stuttering.* Englewood Clifs, NJ: Prentice-Hall, Inc.

If you believe this book has helped you or you wish to help this worthwhile cause, please send a donation to:

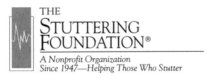

THE
STUTTERING
FOUNDATION®

A Nonprofit Organization
Since 1947—Helping Those Who Stutter

P.O. Box 11749 • Memphis, TN 38111-0749

800-992-9392

www.StutteringHelp.org   www.tartamudez.org
info@stutteringhelp.org

www.StutteringHelp.org

www.tartamudez.org

...DVDs available from the Stuttering Foundation

Sharpening Counseling Skills
with David M. Luterman, D.Ed.

This exciting 3-hour DVD features renowned audiologist and expert counselor, David M. Luterman, D.Ed. Luterman's philosophy of counseling centers around deep listening and silent witnessing of our clients' stories and concerns as we refrain from providing immediate advice, information, or solutions.

Includes subtitles for the hearing impaired   **DVD   No. 9800**

New Dimensions in Parent Counseling
with David M. Luterman, D.Ed.

This unique DVD features master clinician, David Luterman, facilitating a group of parents of children who stutter, using a listening/valuing model of interaction.

This DVD is divided into two parts: *Group Therapy with Parents* (1 hour, 41 minutes) and *Therapists' Review of Parent Session* (1 hour, 27 minutes).

DVD   No. 6400